MAKING SENSE
of DISASTER
MEDICINE

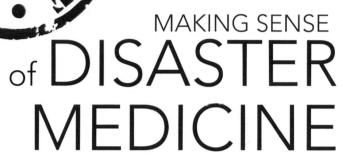

MAKING SENSE
of DISASTER
MEDICINE

A HANDS-ON GUIDE
FOR MEDICS

Dr James IDM Matheson

MBBS, BA (Hons)
Academic Foundation Programme,
Royal Lancaster Infirmary
Catastrophes & Conflict Forum,
Royal Society of Medicine
Faculty of Conflict & Catastrophe Medicine
Society of Apothecaries of London

Professor Alan Hawley OBE QHP

Professor of Disaster Medicine,
Professor of Disaster Studies and
Director of the Disasters and
Resilience Centre
University of Glamorgan

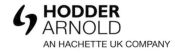
HODDER
ARNOLD
AN HACHETTE UK COMPANY

First published in Great Britain in 2010 by
Hodder Arnold, an imprint of Hodder Education, an Hachette UK company,
338 Euston Road, London NW1 3BH

http://www.hodderarnold.com

© 2010 Hodder Arnold (Publishers) Ltd

Whilst the advice and information in this book are believed to be true and accurate
at the date of going to press, neither the author[s] nor the publisher can accept any
legal responsibility or liability for any errors or omissions that may be made.
In particular, (but without limiting the generality of the preceding disclaimer) every
effort has been made to check drug dosages; however it is still possible that errors
have been missed. Furthermore, dosage schedules are constantly being revised and
new side-effects recognized. For these reasons the reader is strongly urged to
consult the drug companies' printed instructions before administering any of the
drugs recommended in this book.

British Library Cataloguing in Publication Data
A catalogue record for this book is available from the British Library

Library of Congress Cataloging-in-Publication Data
A catalog record for this book is available from the Library of Congress

ISBN-13 978-0-340-96756-0

1 2 3 4 5 6 7 8 9 10

Commissioning Editor: Joanna Koster
Project Editors: Sarah Penny and Stephen Clausard
Production Controller: Jonathan Williams
Cover Design: Amina Dudhia
Copy-editor: Carolyn Holleyman
Indexer: Laurence Errington

Typeset in 11.5/13 pt Chaparral by MPS Limited, a Macmillan Company.
Printed in India for Hodder Education, an Hachette UK Company.

What do you think about this book? Or any other Hodder Arnold title?
Please visit our website: www.hodderarnold.com

To Kathryn and Caroline

Contributors

Dr Laith K Alrubaiy MB ChB, MSc, MRCSEd (A&E)
Specialty Registrar in Core Medical Training,
Ysbyty Gwynedd,
Bangor

Colonel JPG Bolton MB MSc DRCOG MRCGP FFPH L/RAMC
AD Health Surveillance,
Ministry of Defence,
Defence Medical Services Department,
Whitehall, London

Dr Roland MF Gill MBBS, MFOM, MRCGP
Camberley,
Surrey

Mr Jonathan Kaplan MS, ChM, FRCS, DMCC
London

Dr Maria Kett RGN, BA (Hons), PhD
Assistant Director,
Leonard Cheshire Disability and Inclusive Development Centre,
University College London,
London

Pietro D Marghella MS, MA, CEM, FACCP
Professional Lecturer and Director,
Disaster Management for Healthcare Leaders Program,
The George Washington University, Washington, DC
USA

Mr Steven Mannion
Blackpool,
Lancs

Group Captain Aroop Mozumder MSc MBBS MRCGP DRCOG DTM&H DAvMed DMCC RAF
Deputy Assistant Chief of Staff Medical Programmes,
HQ Air Command,
Royal Air Force High Wycombe,
Bucks and Honorary Lecturer
Conflict & Health Unit, London

CONTRIBUTORS

School of Hygiene and Tropical
Medicine, Lecturer and Examiner,
Diploma in Medical Care of
Catastrophes, Society of
Apothecaries of London

Dr Tim O'Dempsey MB ChB,
FRCP, DObs, DCH, DTCH,
DTM&H
Senior Clinical Lecturer in
Tropical Medicine,
Liverpool School of Tropical
Medicine,
Liverpool

Ian Palmer MB ChB, MRCPsych
Professor of Military Psychiatry,
Head of Medical Assessment
Programme, St Thomas' Hospital,
London and Baird Health Centre,
London

Dr Maurice A Ramirez DO, PhD,
BCEM, CNS, CMRO
President/Founder – High Alert,
LLC,
USA

Lieutenant Colonel Ken I Roberts
RAMC
Environmental Health Officer,
Army Medical Directorate,
Former Army Staff College,
Camberley,
Surrey

Lt Colonel David Lloyd Roberts
(Retd) MBE, LLM, Ex ICRC
Delegate
Lockerley,
Hants

Professor Jim Ryan OstJ, MCh,
FRCS, DMCC, FFAEM (Hon)
Emeritus Professor of Conflict
and Catastrophe,
Centre for Trauma, Conflict and
Catastrophe,
St George's, University of London,
London

Dr Daniel K Sokol PhD MSc
MSc MA
Honorary Senior Lecturer in
Medical Ethics, Imperial College,
London

Dr Mark Wilson BSc MBBChir
MRCA FRCS (Surg Neurol)
FIMC(Ed) FRGS
Neurosurgery and
Pre Hospital Care,
Specialist Registrar,
The National Hospital for
Neurology and Neurosurgery and
the Royal London Hospitals,
London

Acknowledgements

With heartfelt thanks to all those who contributed directly to this book and to all those whose hard work and dedication has made a difference in this challenging field of medicine.

List of abbreviations

AADM, American Academy of Disaster Medicine
AAMA, American Academy of Medical Administrators
AAPS, American Association of Physician Specialists
ABODM, American Board of Disaster Medicine
ABPS, American Board of Physician Specialties
ACCP, American College of Contingency Planners
AMREF, African Medical and Research Foundation
AMA, American Medical Association
ARVs, anti-retrovirals
ARDS, adult respiratory distress
ARIs, acute respiratory infections
ACT, artemisinin-based combination therapy
ATLS®, Advanced Trauma Life Support
BASICS, British Association of Immediate Care Specialists
BATLS, Battlefield Advanced Trauma Life Support

C^2, command and control
CBRN, chemical, biological, radiological or nuclear
CHE, complex humanitarian emergency
CI/KR, critical infrastructure and key resource
CMR, crude mortality rate
CMS, Center for Medicare Services
CNA, Center for Naval Analysis
CPR, cardiopulmonary resuscitation
CSF, cerebrospinal fluid
DFID, Department for International Development
DIC, disseminated intravascular coagulation
DMAT, Disaster Medical Assistance Teams
DMCC, Diploma in the Medical Care of Catastrophes
DMORT, Disaster Mortuary Operational Response Teams
DOTS, directly observed treatment clinics
DPOs, Disabled People's Organizations

DPS, delayed primary suture

DSTC, Definitive Surgical Trauma Course

DSTS, definitive surgical trauma skills

EHF, Ebola haemorrhagic fever

EM, emergency medicine

EMAC, Emergency Management Assistance Compact

EMS, Emergency Medical Service

EMTALA, Emergency Medical Treatment and Active Labor Act

EOC, Emergency Operations Center

EPI, Extended Program on Immunization

ERC, Emergency Relief Coordinator

FEBA, forward edge of the battle area

FR, federal response

HC, Humanitarian Coordinator

HCF, Healthcare Facility

HDRO, humanitarian or disaster relief operation

HERC, Hospital Emergency Response Coalition

HHS, Health and Human Services

HPA, Health Protection Agency

HSPD, Homeland Security Presidential Directives

HUS, haemolytic uraemic syndrome

IASC, Inter-Agency Standing Committee

ICRC, International Committee of the Red Cross (and Red Crescent)

ICS, Incident Command System

IDP, internally displaced person

IDRL, International Disaster Response Laws, Rules and Principles

IED, improvised explosive device

IFRC, International Federation of Red Cross and Red Crescent Societies

IMAI, Integrated Management of Adolescent and Adult Illness

IMCI, Integrated Management of Childhood Illness

IMS, Incident Management System

IOM, International Organization for Migration

IOs, international organizations

ITNs, insecticide treated bednets

LBRF, louse-borne relapsing fever

LBT, louse-borne typhus

LP, lumbar puncture

MAC, Management Assistance Compacts

MCH, Maternal and Child Health Clinics

MCI, mass-casualty incidents

MERT, Medical Emergency Response Team

MPI, mass psychogenic illness

MSCC, Medical Surge Capacity and Capability

MSF, Médecins Sans Frontières

MTF, medical treatment facility

MUPS, Multiple Unexplained Physical Symptoms

NaTHNaC, National Travel Health Network and Centre

NATO, North Atlantic Treaty Organization

NDLS, National Disaster Life Support

NDMS, National Disaster Medical System

NGOs, non-governmental organizations

NIMS, National Incident Management System

NMRT, National Medical Response Teams

NPS, National Planning Scenarios

NRP, National Response Plan

NRTS, National Resource Typing System

OCHA, Office for the Coordination of Humanitarian Affairs

ODI, Overseas Development Institute

OHCHR, Office of the High Commissioner for Human Rights

OP, organophosphate

ORS, oral rehydration solution

ORT, oral rehydration therapy

PAR, population at risk

PH, public health

PPE, personal protective equipment

PRTs, Provincial Reconstruction Teams

PTSD, post-traumatic stress disorder

RBCs, red blood cells

RDT, Rapid Diagnostic Test

SARS, severe acute respiratory distress syndrome

SATCOM, satellite communications

SCF-UK, Save the Children Fund-UK

SMART™, Sensitive Membrane Antigen Rapid Test

STIs, sexually transmitted diseases

TCBS, thiosulphate citrate bile salts sucrose

TFCs, therapeutic feeding centres

TMOSAs, temporary medical operations support areas

U5MR, under-5 mortality rate

UNDAC, United Nations Disaster Assessment and Coordination Agency

UNDP, United Nations Development Program

UNHCR, United Nations High Commissioner for Refugees

UNICEF, United Nations International Children's Emergency Fund

UNIFEM, United Nations Development Fund for Women

URL, uniform resource locator

USAID, US Agency for International Development

UXO, unexploded military ordnance

VHFs, viral haemorrhagic fevers

WFP, World Food Programme

WFH, weight for height

WMD, weapons of mass destruction

Contents

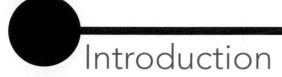

Introduction

James Matheson and Alan Hawley

For some medical students, disaster seems a world away – something that strikes in distant cities or, perhaps, something to be visited in a humanitarian context, sometime in the future, when you are suitably qualified. The reality, sadly, is very different and the truth is that any person may be caught up in some form of disaster at any moment, but the difference for a medical student is that you may have to take a role in the response.

This book is intended to make sense of an exciting and challenging area of medicine and surgery that everyone may be involved in at some point in their lives and that, when that time is upon them, will demand the highest levels of dedication and professionalism, with life or death decision-making taken to a new level, often in the most difficult of environments and with the consequences of failure tragic and immediately apparent.

Disaster Medicine has been around for as long as there have been disasters and people with an interest in their response but now, for the first time, there is an increasing awareness of the broad base of skills required to intervene effectively in catastrophe, of the necessity to formalize and evaluate healthcare professionals' training in the field, to recognize this collection of skills and training in the establishment of the specialty of Disaster Medicine and to ensure the ubiquity of essential disaster response knowledge and skills amongst those who will be called upon to provide that response – in other words, anyone who is medically qualified.

For many years, there has existed a somewhat artificial division in the perception of disasters at home and abroad. International disaster response has suffered from a relative dearth of funding, support and coordination compared with issues which people believed would more likely affect the voting and tax-paying populations of developed countries. Recent weather disasters, especially in the United States and mass casualty incidents in Western countries amidst the 'Global War on Terror' have served to diminish that gap and highlight that many of the same skills and much of the same knowledge is required to act effectively in disaster situations on home soil as in distant lands. For this reason, *Making Sense of Disaster Medicine* covers Disaster Medicine in both an international and domestic context.

● Why me?

The chapters above encompass many threats to the health of your future patients and hopefully demonstrate that, as disaster can strike anywhere at any time, we all should be prepared. Perhaps your interest is deeper, however, and Disaster Medicine is a career path you wish to actively pursue. In some countries such as America you will be able to follow a recognized training route, take exams and qualify and work in Disaster Medicine as a specialty field. Elsewhere you may have to forge your own path, seeking what educational and training opportunities are available and hunting out specialist roles in which you can apply the skills you learn.

One such area is in humanitarian work with its short-term disaster response and longer term emergency missions. Whatever your professional area of interest, almost every specialty can make a useful impact in some part of the world when carefully applied. Humanitarian work, however, is not something which should or even can be undertaken lightly. Modern Non-Governmental Organizations (NGOs) require evidence of your training and experience before they will allow you to work on their behalf in an arena where standards and accountability are increasingly to the fore. If you have ideas of working overseas in the future you will have to start preparing yourself now or risk losing out on some great opportunities.

● Getting involved

Disaster Medicine may appear like a specialty interest it is hard to penetrate into at the very start of your medical learning, but appearances can be deceptive. People with an interest in the field like to share their knowledge and enthusiasm for the subject and this offers a number of great opportunities to get yourself involved.

Look out for conferences

Scan the internet and hospital and medical school noticeboards for the groups that work in the field and when they plan to get together. You'll hear interesting and inspirational lectures and, perhaps most importantly, meet the people who work in the area who can advise you on how and why to join the cause.

Become one of the gang

With concerns about legal liability, many large NGOs will hesitate to take medical students into the field, especially into hazardous areas. If you are well-informed, appropriately trained and sensible, however, some will and it always helps if you are well-known to the people in question. Some NGOs run internship programmes with attachments split between their home offices and projects in the fields. Others give you the opportunity to become a 'friend of' the charity – this may only involve fundraising and helping out at events, but it will demonstrate your commitment, allow you to meet relevant people and learn more about the work, all of which will show you in a good light when it comes to selection for missions. Look for organizations that have an academic interest in the field of Disaster Medicine – in the UK, the Royal Society of Medicine's Catastrophes and Conflict Forum (www.rsm.ac.uk)

and the Society of Apothecaries' Faculty of Conflict and Catastrophe Medicine (www.apothecaries.org) are examples and both have student representative posts.

Be ready for disaster at home

Read your hospital's major incident plan. Most plans have a role for students within them as students are numerous, enthusiastic and readily available – you are a useful resource in times of over-stretch. Make sure you can carry out your role in the plan. Often this will be as a runner – perhaps not the most glamorous sounding position but vital – make sure you know your way around the whole hospital, not just the wards you've visited on attachment. If you are in more senior years do not be surprised if you have a more clinical role in disaster management. If you can clerk patients on the ward you may be required to assist when the surge of patients threatens to overwhelm available staff on the floor. Hospitals must rehearse their major incident plans regularly. Find out when the next practice is and volunteer your services to whoever is in charge. Remember that disaster may strike on your way to work – in the street or on the bus or underground. You need to be able to respond usefully – get yourself First Aid trained if your medical school does not adequately train you, and sign up to be an observer at an Advanced Trauma Life Support course near you. If you can't observe on such courses they always need people to role play casualties and this is a better learning experience than nothing at all.

Get trained and educated

As mentioned above, selection for disaster work at home or abroad can be as competitive as applying for training in the most over-subscribed medical and surgical specialties and, as with any such challenge, the key is to be properly prepared. The organization you wish to work with will want to be assured that you know what you're doing and have the appropriate skills to work, often unsupported, many miles from your usual medical team and its comforts back home. This means education and courses. Reading this book is a good start, and follow up on its recommended reading lists. Check out what is available (see Chapter 5 for details) but be careful you don't end up paying for courses that your NGO will provide for free. In the United States, look at taking the Disaster Life Support courses – 'basic' and 'advanced' can be done as a student and the 'core' qualification is now available online. Of UK courses, the Diploma in Tropical Medicine and Diploma in the Medical Care of Catastrophes (DMCC) will stand you in good stead for both selection and deployment on mission. These are both postgraduate diplomas (although you can attend the DMCC course as a student, potentially at a discounted rate) but there are undergraduate opportunities as well. Many universities run disaster or humanitarian-related courses and an increasing number of medical schools have established or are developing intercalated degrees with a higher clinical content such as the intercalated BSc in Leadership in Disaster Medicine at St George's, University of London. The better your understanding of the complexities of disaster work, the more likely you are to be selected and the better job you'll do once you get there.

Get experience

One of the first things large aid organizations ask for is experience in the field. They want to know that you know what you're letting yourself in for and if you can be relied upon to live and work in this particular environment. It is something of a vicious circle that you need experience to get in the door of the organizations that can give you the necessary experience, but there are ways around this. First, be sure to use your elective suitably (see below) – this may not be sufficient for all organizations but it is a good start. It can be tricky as a medical student or junior doctor to find someone who thinks your skills are adequate to be useful and to get sufficient leave to go overseas, but some organizations are more tailored towards this. Check out your hospital's international healthcare links – your hospital should be linked with one in the developing world and should provide opportunities for staff and students to gain experience overseas and become involved with the running of the link, providing useful administrative and logistic experience for work in the field. If your hospital doesn't have a link then set one up – this is a simple process, which if done correctly (see www.thet.org for the Tropical Health and Education Trust) can have a useful global health impact and give you great experience along the way.

Get involved in research

Your medical school will have research interests all over the world and some of these will have a Disaster Medicine application. Approach the Infectious Diseases department as a good start – you may be able to contribute usefully and there may be opportunities to gain experience working abroad. Conferences are another good place to meet people with research interests in the field and ask to join their team. Research in Disaster Medicine is presently notably lacking, but is a field which must be expanded and built upon to take the specialty forward on a scientific basis in the future.

Use your elective

If you have an interest in Disaster Medicine, you will probably not want to spend your elective on the wards in your local hospital. The options for elective are numerous, but in Disaster Medicine consider either using the time to qualify and gain experience in a country where Disaster Medicine is established such as the US, or gain experience working in the developing world where the population is vulnerable to catastrophe or experiencing more long-term healthcare emergencies. Try to gain a new perspective in this field rather than simply following the ward round in a foreign hospital as you might back home. Perhaps you could even combine the two experiences with time spent in each, very different environment and make a comparison of what you see. If you are doing something out of the ordinary you will find it easier to attract funding (and prizes) for your project. You may wish to work in conflict areas in the future but these may not be the best places to learn the business. Don't go anywhere where you're not capable of looking after yourself – you're no help to anyone as a casualty or if you are kidnapped. Electives are a wonderful opportunity and Chapter 14 will give you lots of help finding the right elective for you.

Share what you learn

There are an increasing number of publications with an interest in Disaster Medicine. The online *Lancet* publication, www.TheLancetStudent.com and the journal *Medicine, Conflict and Survival* are two examples which will publish high quality submissions from students. The *Student BMJ* and *Student BMA News* will publish elective reports and you can even gain prizes for them. So read up on your area of interest, speak to the people involved in it, write it up and share what you have learned with other students interested in the field. As a student with a decent amount of spare time, you have much to offer (this book was co-edited by a medical student). As well as providing a service you will build up a list of publications demonstrating your interest and commitment which will serve you well when applying for positions with a Disaster Medicine role.

● Leadership in Disaster Medicine

Medicine, for all its talk of the importance of the team, retains a fairly hierarchical structure and, as a medical student, you may feel very much at the bottom of it. Disaster Medicine is a field which relies enormously on good leadership, appropriately applied and, given the particular challenges of the work, even more so than in the hospital's day to day life. It is also a nascent field in most parts of the world where you, if you have something to offer, can take a role, become a driving force and shape the direction and impact of Disaster Medicine in the future.

Leadership is not for everyone but, having embarked upon a medical career, as the doctor in the team you may well be looked upon to take the lead and, in Disaster Medicine, in particularly trying circumstances. Leadership in these circumstances is about much more than just clinical decision-making. It will involve ethical decision-making which may take great moral courage. A certain amount of physical courage may be involved also. You will have to look after your patients who may number in the thousands, your team who will be over-stretched and under-resourced and yourself, who will have to live with the consequences of each decision you make. If this sounds horrendous to you, these are challenges you must overcome; if it sounds like just what you've been looking for, you may be a leader in the making. Research the field, find out what needs doing and get down to work, recruiting others to join you. This is a part of medicine where you can really make a difference.

● The future

Disaster Medicine is a constantly evolving field. Natural disasters are increasing in frequency and, due to the spread of the human population to ever more precarious parts of the planet, increasing in impact. Ongoing conflict has raised the profile of disasters at home and diverted funding into their response. Disaster Medicine has become established as a medical specialty in some parts of the developed world and now, more than ever, the need and the opportunity to develop it universally are apparent. It is clear that what was once the preserve of a selected few, in public health disaster planning and on the front line in emergency medicine, must now become core skills of every physician in order to competently and professionally attend to the demands of disaster response. As societies we have a duty of care to our populations to ensure these services are available just as, as doctors, we have a duty of care to our patients when disaster strikes them. This exciting and challenging field of medicine is about to take a new course and one in which you can play an important role.

Since this chapter was written there have been a number of headline disasters and the response to them has brought some interesting developments. Earthquakes have been prominent in the news with large events in Chile, Haiti and China. Haiti, in particular, has provided a news focus, partly perhaps because, as with the Asian tsunami, it occurred in a popular western holiday destination.

Haiti once again highlighted issues, positive and negative, about international disaster response. For a period of time public interest was transfixed on this little area of the world. The earthquake itself was dramatic but its impact was magnified by the vulnerability of the population it affected. Much of the nation's capital was destroyed – a poor country, little had been invested in its infrastructure and building standards had not been enforced. Much of Haiti's population lived on the brink of disaster on a daily basis and with the earthquake regular incomes were lost, sources of clean water disrupted and what little law and order there had been vanished.

The international response was rapid by response standards and was characterized, as many times previously, by the military taking the lead and civilian agencies following. From the UK, our firemen arrived swiftly in a search and rescue capacity but found themselves frustrated at how little medical aid was in place. The press, as ever highly mobile, were quick to point out that, even when the international response was well underway, they only had to go a very short distance from the airport to see where its reach ended. There was progress, however, with a potential forerunner of a national surgical response to disaster deploying in coordination with one of UK's main aid agencies. Haiti, at once, showed the potential for major international responses but also their limitations. We have a long way to go to maximize the impact that international concern can translate into but Haiti may have shown a new direction in the UK's role in disaster response.

We hope that *Making Sense of Disaster Medicine* will give you a clearer understanding of key areas of Disaster Medicine and their importance and help you develop your role in disaster response in the future.

Disaster medicine: Evolution of a specialty

Maurice A. Ramirez

Introduction

Today there is a need to effectively organize and coordinate disaster planning, action and the application of knowledge and understanding. This need transcends all considerations and professions and especially healthcare. We must be prepared, especially physicians, in responding to all types of disasters for the public good and that of the nation. It is well-known that most physicians lack disaster medical training and there is currently a nationwide shortage of appropriately trained physicians to respond to national disaster. Regulatory and Government agencies have recognized disaster preparedness as a major healthcare need.

Disaster medicine as a specialty and mindset was not only a reaction from September 11, 2001, but to the numerous subsequent events that seemed to all too quickly follow: random anthrax attacks in the weeks afterwards, the severe acute respiratory distress syndrome (SARS) outbreak in pockets of the world, the blackout in the summer of 2003 that took the power out in New York City and surrounding cities and states, the December 26, 2004 Indian Ocean tsunami, the Pakistan earthquake of 2005, a tumultuous hurricane season in 2005 culminating with the arrival of Hurricane Katrina and, of course, terrorist attacks throughout the world including Spain, England, Bangladesh and Bali – all against a backdrop of conflict in Afghanistan and Iraq.

● Scope of practice

Disaster Medicine is the area of healthcare specialization serving the dual areas of providing medical care to disaster survivors and providing medically related disaster preparation, disaster planning, disaster response and disaster recovery leadership throughout the disaster life cycle.

Disaster Medicine specialists provide insight, guidance and expertise on the principles and practice of medicine both in the disaster impact area and healthcare evacuation-receiving facilities to emergency management professionals, hospitals, healthcare facilities, communities and governments. The Disaster Medicine specialist is the liaison between and partner to the medical contingency planner, the emergency management professional, the incident command system, government and policy makers.

Internationally, Disaster Medicine specialists must demonstrate competency in areas of disaster healthcare and emergency management including but not limited to:

- disaster behavioural health
- disaster law
- disaster planning
- disaster preparation
- disaster recovery
- disaster response
- disaster scene safety
- emergency management
- emergency operations (Incident Command)
- forensics and disaster
- medical consequences of disaster
- medical consequences of terrorism

- medical contingency planning
- medical decontamination
- medical implications of disaster
- medical implications of terrorism
- medical planning and preparation for disaster
- medical planning and preparation for terrorism
- medical recovery from disaster
- medical recovery from terrorism
- medical response to disaster
- medical response to terrorism
- medical response to weapons of mass destruction
- medical surge, surge capacity and triage
- psychosocial implications of disaster
- psychosocial implications of terrorism
- psychosocial triage.

Complicating the role of the Disaster Medicine specialist is that fact that each of these areas of function must be customized for the culture, country, region and municipality where the Disaster Medicine specialist practises. Fortunately, there are principles common to the practice of disaster medicine worldwide and even across these areas of function and subspecialization.

Disaster Medicine is unique among the medical specialties in that the Disaster Medicine specialist does not practise the full scope of the specialty everyday. Indeed, the Disaster Medicine specialist hopes to never practice the full scope of skills required for board certification. Like the specialists in public health, environmental medicine and occupational medicine, however, Disaster Medicine specialists engage in the development and modification of public and private policy, legislation and regulation as it relates to disaster preparation, disaster planning, disaster education, disaster response and disaster recovery.

Within the United States of America, the specialty of Disaster Medicine fulfils the requirements set by Homeland Security

Presidential Directives (HSPD), the National Response Plan (NRP), the National Incident Management System (NIMS), the National Resource Typing System (NRTS) and the NIMS Implementation Plan for Hospitals and Healthcare Facilities. Similar requirements exist within the United Kingdom and the nascent specialty of Disaster Medicine in Great Britain will address these and future needs while serving as a model for the rest of Europe.

 LEARNING POINTS

Definitions

Disaster healthcare – Defined by the HSPDs as the provision of healthcare services by healthcare professionals to disaster survivors and disaster responders both in a disaster impact area and healthcare evacuation-receiving facilities throughout the disaster life cycle (for details of HSPDs see Further reading).

Disaster behavioural health – Deals with the capability of disaster responders to perform optimally and for disaster survivors to maintain or rapidly restore function, when faced with the threat or actual impact of disasters and extreme events (Shultz *et al.*, 2006).

Disaster law – Deals with the legal ramifications of disaster planning, preparedness, response and recovery, including but not limited to financial recovery, public and private liability, property abatement and condemnation.

Disaster life cycle – The time line for disaster events beginning with the period between disasters (Interphase), progressing through the disaster event and the disaster response and culminating in the disaster recovery. Interphase begins at the end of the last disaster recovery and ends at the onset of the next disaster event. The disaster event begins when the event occurs and ends when the immediate event subsides. The disaster response begins when the event occurs and ends when acute disaster response services are no longer needed. Disaster recovery also begins with the disaster response and continues until the affected area is returned to the pre-event condition (Marghella, 2007).

Disaster planning – The act of devising a methodology for dealing with a disaster event, especially one with the potential to occur suddenly and cause great injury and/or loss of life, damage and hardship. Disaster planning occurs during the disaster interphase (Marghella, 2007).

Disaster preparation – The act of practising and implementing the plan for dealing with a disaster event before an event occurs, especially one with the potential to occur suddenly and cause great injury and/or loss of life, damage and hardship. Disaster preparation occurs during the disaster interphase (Marghella, 2007).

Disaster recovery – The restoration or return to the former or better state or condition preceding a disaster event (i.e. status quo ante, the state of affairs that existed previously). Disaster recovery is the fourth phase of the disaster life cycle (Marghella, 2007).

Disaster response – The ability to answer the intense challenges posed by a disaster event. Disaster response is the third phase of the disaster life cycle (Marghella, 2007).

Medical contingency planning – The act of devising a methodology for meeting the medical requirements of a population affected by a disaster event (Marghella, 2007).

Medical surge – An influx of patients (physical casualties and psychological casualties), bystanders, visitors, family members, media and individuals searching for the missing who present to a hospital or healthcare facility for treatment, information and/or shelter as a result of a disaster (Shultz *et al.*, 2006).

Surge capacity – The ability to manage a sudden, unexpected increase in patient volume that would otherwise severely challenge or exceed the current capacity of the healthcare system (Barbera and McIntyre, 2003).

Medical triage – The separation of patients based on severity of injury or illness in light of available resources (see Surge, Sort, Support Lecture Series in Further reading).

Psychosocial triage – The separation of patients based on the severity of psychological injury or impact in light of available resources (as above).

● History

The term 'Disaster Medicine' first appeared in the medical lexicon in the post World War II era. Although coined by former and current military physicians who had served in World War II, the term did not refer to the care of military casualties, or nuclear war victims, but to the need to provide care to the survivors of natural disasters and the not yet distant memory of the 1917–18 influenza pandemic.

The term 'Disaster Medicine' would continue to appear sporadically in both the medical and popular press until the 1980s when the first concerted efforts to organize a medical response corps for disasters grew into the National Disaster Medical System. Simultaneously came the formation of a disaster and emergency medicine discussion and study group under the American Medical Association (AMA) in the United States as well as groups in Great Britain, Israel and other countries. By the time Hurricane Andrew struck Florida in 1992, the concept of Disaster Medicine was entrenched in public and governmental consciousness. Although training and fellowships in Disaster Medicine or related topics began graduating specialists in Europe and the United States as early as the 1980s, it would not be until 2003 that the medical community would embrace the need for the new specialty.

Throughout this period, incomplete and faltering medical responses to disaster events made it increasingly apparent that emergency management organizations at all levels of government were in need of a mechanism to identify qualified physicians in the face of a global upturn in the rate of natural and man-made disasters. Many physicians who volunteer at disasters have minimal knowledge of Disaster Medicine and often pose a hazard to themselves and the response effort because they have little or no field response training. It was against this backdrop that the American Academy of Disaster Medicine (AADM) and the American Board of Disaster Medicine (ABODM) were formed as the first specialty organizations dedicated solely to scholarly exchange and education in Disaster Medicine as well as the development of an examination demonstrating excellence towards board certification in this new specialty.

● Time line

1812 – Napoleonic wars give rise to the military medical practice of triage in an effort to sort wounded soldiers into those to receive medical treatment and return to battle and those whose injuries are non-survivable. Dominique-Jean Larrey, a surgeon in the French Emperor's army, conceived the idea of taking care of the wounded on the battlefield, and also created the concept of ambulances, collecting the wounded in horse-drawn wagons and taking them to military hospitals.

1863 – International Red Cross founded in Geneva, Switzerland.

1873 – Clara Barton organizes the American Red Cross during the American Civil War.

1937 – President Franklin Roosevelt makes a public request by commercial radio for medical aid following a natural gas explosion in New London, Texas. This is the first presidential request for disaster medical assistance in United States history.

1955 – Colonel Karl H. Houghton, MD's address to a convention of military surgeons, introducing the concept of 'Disaster Medicine' is reported in the *Reno Evening Gazette*.

1959 – Colonel Joseph R. Schaeffer, MD reflecting the growing national concern over nuclear attacks on the United States civilian population initiates training for civilian physicians in the treatment of mass casualties for the effects of weapons of mass destruction creating the concept of medical surge capacity.

1961 – The AMA, the American Hospital Association, the American College of Surgeons, the United States Public Health Service, the United States Office of Civil Defense and the Department of Health, Education and Welfare join Dr Schaeffer in advancing civilian physician training for mass casualty and weapons of mass destruction treatment.

1962 – The North Atlantic Treaty Organization (NATO) publishes an official Disaster Medicine manual edited by Dr Schaeffer.

1984 – The United States Public Health Service forms the first federal disaster medical response team in Washington, DC designated PHS-1.

1986 – The Unites States Public Health System creates the National Disaster Medical System (NDMS) to provide disaster healthcare through National Medical Response Teams (NMRT), Disaster Medical Assistance Teams (DMAT) and Disaster Mortuary Operational Response Teams (DMORT). PH-1 becomes the first DMAT team.

1986 – A disaster medical response discussion group is created by NDMS team members and emergency medicine organizations in the United States. Healthcare professionals worldwide join the discussion group.

1989 – The University of New Mexico creates the Center for Disaster Medicine, the first such medical centre of excellence in the United States. Elsewhere in the world, similar centers are created at universities in London, Paris, Brussels and Bordeaux.

1992 – Hurricane Andrew, a category 5 hurricane strikes south Florida destroying the city of Homestead, Florida and initiating the largest disaster healthcare response to date.

1993 – On February 26, 1993 at 12.17, a Ryder truck filled with 1500 pounds (680 kg) of explosives was planted by Ramzi Yousef and detonated in the underground garage of the North Tower, opening a 100 foot (30 m) hole through five sublevels of concrete leaving six people dead and 50 000 other workers and visitors gasping for air in the shafts of the 110-story towers. The first World Trade Center bombing is also the first terrorist attack on United States soil since World War II and increases interest in specialized education on the treatment of weapons of mass destruction and terrorism response for civilian physicians.

1995 – Timothy McVey perpetrates the Oklahoma City bombing on April 19, 1995, at 09.01 local time destroying the Alfred P. Murrah Federal Building, a Federal government of the United States government office complex. The attack claimed 168 lives and raised the spectre of domestic terrorism as a medical response concern for the United States.

1998 – The American College of Contingency Planners (ACCP) is formed by the American Academy of Medical Administrators (AAMA) to provide certification and scholarly study in the area of medical contingency planning and healthcare disaster planning.

2001 – The September 11, 2001 attacks on the World Trade Center and the Pentagon is the largest loss of life resulting from an attack on American targets on United States soil since Pearl Harbor. As a result, the need for Disaster Medicine is galvanized worldwide.

2003 – The American Medical Association in conjunction with the Medical College of Georgia and the University of Texas debut the National Disaster Life Support (NDLS) training programme providing the first national certification in disaster medicine skills and education. NDLS training would later be referred to as 'the cardiopulmonary resuscitation (CPR) of the twenty-first century'.

2003 – In February, 2003 the American Association of Physician Specialists (AAPS) appoints an expert panel to explore the question of whether Disaster Medicine qualifies as a medical specialty.

2004 – In February, 2004 the AAPS reports to the American Board of Physician Specialties (ABPS) that the expert panel, supported by the available literature and recent HSPDs has determined that there is a sufficient body of unique knowledge in Disaster Medicine to designate the field as a discrete specialty. ABPS empanels a board of certification to determine if board certification is appropriate in this new specialty.

2004 – On April 28, 2004, President Bush issues HSPD-10, also known as the plan for Biodefense for the twenty-first century, which calls for healthcare to implement surveillance and response capabilities to combat the threat of terrorism.

2004 – Hurricanes Charlie, Francis, Ivan and Jeanne batter the state of Florida resulting in the largest disaster medical response since Hurricane Andrew.

2005 – Hurricane Katrina batters the Gulf Coast of the United States destroying multiple coastal cities. For the first time in NDMS history, the entire NDMS system is deployed for a single disaster medical response. Among the many lessons learned in field operations following Hurricane Katrina are the need for cellular autonomy under a central incident command structure and the creation of continuous integrated triage for the management of massive patient surge. The lessons learned in the Hurricane Katrina response would be applied less than a month later following Hurricane Rita and again following Hurricane Wilma and the Indonesian tsunami.

2005 – In late October, 2005, the American Board of Disaster Medicine (ABODM) and the American Academy of Disaster Medicine (AADM) were formed for scholarly study, discussion and exchange in the field of Disaster Medicine as well as to oversee board certification.

2006 – In June, the Institute of Medicine published three reports on the state of emergency healthcare in the United States. Among the condemnations of emergency care is the lack of substantial improvement in disaster preparedness or 'cross silo' coordination.

2006 – On September 17, the NIMS Integration Center publishes the NIMS Implementation Plan for Hospitals and Healthcare establishing a September 30, 2007 deadline for all hospitals and healthcare facilities to be 'NIMS compliant'.

2007 – On January 31, President Bush issues HSPD-18 calling for the development and deployment of medical countermeasures against weapons of mass destruction.

2007 – On October 18, 2007, President Bush issues HSPD-21 outlining an augmented plan for public health and disaster medical preparedness. HSPD-21 specifically calls for the creation of the discipline of 'disaster healthcare' using the accepted definition of 'Disaster Medicine'. HSPD-21 also calls on the Secretary of Health and Human Services (HHS) to use 'economic incentives' including the Center for Medicare Services (CMS) to induce private medical organizations, hospitals and healthcare facilities to implement disaster healthcare programmes and medical disaster preparedness programmes.

● Common principles and skills for the Disaster Medicine specialist

Reactive and proactive triage

Reactive triage in the setting of Disaster Medicine is synonymous with mass casualty medical triage and represents the adaptation of care priorities in reaction to the mass casualty event. Reactive triage in this setting is also known as **'Continuous integrated triage'** (Fig. 1.1). Proactive triage is the application of medical triage principles to logistical and operational processes

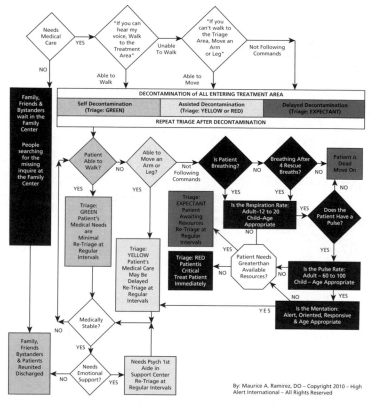

Fig. 1.1 Integrated triage.

during the planning and preparation stage of the disaster life cycle. Proactive triage is a form of process analysis and resource allocation; also known as **'Business triage'**.

Continuous integrated triage

The concept of resource-based decision-making would seem to be basic to the practice of medicine and especially Disaster Medicine. The reality is that, in most industrialized nations, medical care decisions are not resource-based, they are emotionally based. Unfortunately more and more in a world now awakened to the dual threats of terrorism and natural disaster, resource-based decision-making, i.e. triage, is becoming a skill not only needed but often found lacking.

> **PEARL OF WISDOM**
>
> The primary principle to bear in mind regarding triage is that triage is an ongoing process, with patients receiving repeated evaluation and prioritization during the entire time that a person is seeking and receiving medical care from the moment they first approach the medical unit until the moment that they finally leave the care environment.

Triage as a process is also integrated, using the best and most efficient of the available triage methods, beginning with gross observations:

- Can the patient walk?
- Do they follow commands?
- Do they know who they are, where they are and why they are here?

Progressing to basic physiology:

- Are they breathing?
- Do they have a pulse?
- Can they follow commands?

And finally including more detailed information:

- Why was the patient actually brought for care?
- What happened to them?
- What are their needs?
- What are their expectations?

Unfortunately most triage ends when the last question is answered. In the daily practice of triage in the emergency room and in medical practice the process need go no further.

THINKING POINT

For triage to work in the mass casualty environment reactively (and in the planning environment proactively), triage processes must be integrated into our minds and into our moment-to-moment medical practice.

At first glance, the thinking point challenge would seem to be a minor problem; something that can easily be corrected with a small amount of practice. Reality demonstrates a far different truth. As this form of continuous integrated triage was first taught across the United States of America, a disturbing trend was discovered: while healthcare providers readily embraced the idea of continuously reassessing their patients (in fact nurses have done this for decades) the idea of re-categorizing patients, particularly those in the most dire need, was still greatly emotionally laden (Ramirez, 2007).

HAZARD

There are reports now surfacing of facilities that refuse to categorize any patient as anything less than absolutely critical until a full physical examination, laboratory evaluations and even CT scans have been done. At these institutions the entire concept of triage, sorting the masses so that the most good can be done for the most people, has been lost. They are not performing triage. They are jumping straight into treatment (see Further reading).

Of even greater concern are a few isolated reports of facilities refusing to allow providers to bypass patients for whom there are not resources immediately available. These are most often referred to as 'black tag' patients or those who are 'expectant', and they are those who require more resources than are available and prudent to utilize for one person at this time. They are heartrending for the healthcare provider, because under different circumstances these patients are people who could be treated and saved. The problem is that healthcare professionals today do not understand that, although set aside, these patients are not abandoned.

THINKING POINT

A 'black tag' is not a death warrant. It is not a 'Do Not Resuscitate' order. It is not an order to abandon all care. 'Expectant patients' still receive comfort care, compassion, and human dignity. They are still continuously re-triaged and as resources become available, they are brought back into the treatment mix.

When victim counts soar, fatalities soar as well. This is when the Disaster Medicine professional must make decisions. These are the decisions that fall to the professional handling triage.

CASE STUDY

Hurricane Katrina
In the Louis Armstrong International Airport in New Orleans, following Hurricane Katrina during the first five horrendous days of triage and treatment of tens of

thousands of patients and evacuees, only 38 individuals were placed in the expectant category. Of these 38, 36 were ultimately re-triaged, treated, stabilized and sent on to hospitals outside of the state of Louisiana. All 36 of these individuals survived those harrowing days in the airport. Two people did die. In both cases these individuals already had known terminal disease. They were in fact in hospice care before the hurricane. One of these brave souls even refused transportation to allow somebody who had a 'better chance' to go ahead of them. These two 'expectant patients' died in the airport. At the time that they died they were the only two people left in the expectant treatment area. They each had their own nurse provided by the responders at the facility. Each of them had family members at their bedside and local volunteers to sit with them (Shultz *et al.*, 2006).

In the case of each of these individuals, after they died their families commented that they had received better care in the Louis Armstrong International Airport following a hurricane than they would have received at home; not because hospice was in any way incapable but because in the airport they each had their own nurse. Doctors saw them four times a day. They each had their own volunteer and their family crowded around them (Shultz *et al.*, 2006).

Again, we see that the dreaded 'black tag' given to the expectant patient is not a death warrant. It is an opportunity for the healthcare professionals and that patient to do the most human thing possible when part of an overwhelming situation – it is an opportunity to think about others first.

Business triage

Business triage is a system of process analysis and resource allocation for resource-limited business environments both within and outside the healthcare industry. Applying business triage, it is possible to identify and concentrate resources on those outcomes which are most important to mission success.

The first step in each of these triage techniques is to identify and categorize desired outcomes – Critical/Essential, Urgent/Important and Supportive/Optional. Once the outcomes are classified into these categories, identify the processes that result in the desired outcomes. Once the processes are identified, they too must be categorized as above. Next the resources needed for each process are identified and categorized.

Essential/Critical Outcomes are fully supported first with all available resources, then Urgent/Important and finally Supportive/Optional. The use of business triage eliminates the emotionally based tendency to direct resources to the area of greatest consumption or most imminent outage.

This system of proactive triage is particularly useful for the healthcare professional given their familiarity with medical decision-making and medical (reactive) triage principles and represents a unique skill that the Disaster Medicine specialist brings to the disaster preparation and disaster planning process.

● Core competencies

An area of medical specialization is defined by a body of unique knowledge and skills required by practitioners in that field. In February 2003, prior to formation of the AADM and ABODM, AAPS commissioned an expert panel to undertake a scholarly review of the literature and survey the recognized experts in disaster management, emergency management, medical contingency planning, emergency medicine, public health, disaster behavioural health and military medicine to determine if such a unique body of knowledge and skills existed. By February of 2004 it was determined that the majority of experts, supported by the available literature, agreed that there is a unique body of core knowledge and skills to define the specialty of Disaster Medicine and a broader body of knowledge needed by all healthcare practitioners responding to a disaster event.

Beginning in February 2004 through October 2005 further research was completed to compile this body of unique knowledge into a Core Competencies document. By January of 2005, it was evident that the National Disaster Life Support Educational Consortium and the AMA were similarly compiling the body of knowledge needed by all healthcare professionals responding to disasters. As the purpose of the AAPS Disaster Medicine Core Competencies is to define the core body of knowledge required to demonstrate proficiency in Disaster Medicine towards Board Certification in the specialty, the Core Competency document reflects that bias.

Once the Core Competency document was drafted, the AADM through the ABODM reviewed the document against the existing literature and again solicited expert opinion regarding the Domains of Competence and Areas of Competency contained in the document. The Core Competencies were formatted using a modified Bloom's Taxonomy based on the fact that all the competencies contained therein are aimed at the physician leader who seeks to demonstrate excellence in the field of Disaster Medicine. The Core Competencies committee, the AADM and the ABODM recognize that many, but not all the competencies contained in the Core Competencies document are also needed by all healthcare professionals responding to disasters. The final draft document was published in February of 2006 and last revised in April of 2007 (see Tables 1.1a and 1.1b).

Simultaneously, but independently, an expert working group of the AMA, based on a literature review, identified a set of cross-cutting, evidence-based competencies, applicable to all potential health system disaster responders. The working group also identified important potential learning gaps, such as in public health law, ethics, risk communication, cultural

Table 1.1a American Association of Physician Specialists (AAPS) Domains of Competency

	Domain number
Incident Command System: Works as a member of the disaster team under the structure of the Incident Command System.	1
Preparation and Mitigation: Participates in planning for disaster preparation and mitigation.	2
Triage: Performs triage as appropriate in the disaster environment.	3
Decontamination/PPE: Follows appropriate decontamination principles and procedures.	4
Public Health and Safety: Advises on and coordinates aspects of public health and safety throughout the disaster life cycle.	5
Psychosocial Considerations: Provides psychosocial support as appropriate throughout the disaster life cycle.	6
Support/Assistance: Works with various groups and organizations (governmental, community, non-governmental, volunteers) to optimize support for disaster planning, response, and recovery.	7
Communication/Documentation: Maintains necessary communication and documentation.	8
Regulatory/Legal/Ethical Principles: Complies with regulatory and legal as well as accepted moral and ethical principles.	9
Assessment and Treatment: Assesses and treats injuries resulting from natural/non-natural and incidental/intentional causes in a variety of environments (urban, rural, austere).	10
Pathology	11

PPE, personal protection equipment.

competence, mass fatality management, forensics, contingency planning and response and crisis leadership. In addition, it was determined that competencies needed to be comprehensive to ensure they address individuals and populations who may be more vulnerable to adverse health effects in a disaster (e.g. children, pregnant women, frail elderly, disabled persons). As a result, a new conceptual educational model was proposed,

Table 1.1b American Association of Physician Specialists (AAPS) Core Competencies

	Competency number
Incident Command System: Participates as a member of the disaster team under the structure of the Incident Command System.	1
Understands the structure of the Incident Command System (Logistics-Operational-Financing-Planning): knows the organization of the Emergency Operations Center, the ICS table of organization and the role and responsibilities of the public information officer (PIO), the safety officer, incident commander, liaison officer, communications, and related topics such as NIMS and HEICS; understands the chain of command and chain of responsibility.	1.1
Understands basic concepts related to command location, gathering sites (Red, Yellow, Green), site control, span of control, site safety, stockpile issues (strategic, primary loads, local/community, pharmacy), contracting/resupply.	1.2
Understands how to establish the site perimeter and subdivide into hot, warm and cold zones as appropriate.	1.3
Preparation and Mitigation: Participates in planning for disaster preparation and mitigation.	2
Has the knowledge and skills to serve in a major planning role in areas related to PHS, immunization, health/nutrition, sanitation/water, special populations (e.g. paediatrics, geriatric, mobility issues, pregnancy).	2.1
Has the knowledge and skills to participate in the setup and supervision of disaster planning/exercises/training in a variety of settings (hospitals, community/schools, regional/state, federal, personal).	2.2
Understands basic concepts of credentialing/education, funding/granting, interagency agreements (mutual aid, EMTALA Transfer), resupply contracting, EMS/alternate transportation, shelters.	2.3
Triage: Performs triage as appropriate in the disaster environment.	3
Understands the role and implementation of triage and can differentiate between disaster and non-disaster triage.	3.1
Has basic operational knowledge of the major disaster triage systems (i.e. START/PRM, JumpSTART, MASS) and can use one of these methods to perform triage that results in appropriate tags and records.	3.2
Decontamination/PPE: Follows appropriate decontamination principles and procedures.	4
Knows what comprises levels A, B, C, and D and can determine the level of PPE required for each.	4.1
Has the knowledge and skills to perform Level C decontamination.	4.2

| Public Health and Safety: Advises on and coordinates aspects of public health and safety throughout the disaster life cycle. | 5 |

Has knowledge and skills in **environmental** aspects of public health and safety, including sanitation, water, nutrition, immunization, voluntary and compulsory evacuation, scene control, weather monitoring and modelling, shelters, dispersion modelling and monitoring.   5.1

Has knowledge and skills in aspects of public health and safety related to **disease**, including immunization/prophylaxis, surveillance/epidemiology, emerging disease modelling, vector control, lab/path services, treatment.   5.2

Has knowledge and skills related to **complex humanitarian disaster**, including issues related to pharmacy services, refugee/evacuees, physical recovery, special populations, morgue services.   5.3

Psychosocial Considerations: Provides psychosocial support as appropriate throughout the disaster life cycle.   6

Can recognize, assess, and develop a treatment plan for incident-related stress for responders and their team members and families as well as community/victims through the disaster life cycle.   6.1

Understands the role of groups such as clergy, NGOs, volunteers, and grief counsellors in Critical Incident Stress Management (CISM) and Psychological First Aid (PFA).   6.2

Understands the psychosocial needs of special populations, especially paediatric.   6.3

Support/Assistance: Works with various groups and organizations (governmental, community, non-governmental, volunteers) to optimize support for disaster planning, response, and recovery.   7

Understands the roles and the integration of groups such as the following: NDMS (DMORTs/ME, IMSURTS, DMAT, VMAT, NMRT), Community (Law Enforcement, Fire/Rescue, EMS, Public Works), NGOs, Military/National Guard/Coast Guard, FEMA, FBI, CERTs, Public Health personnel, CDC, USAMRICD, WMD-CSTs, Poison Control, vendors, and other specialists (e.g. medical, nuclear).   7.1

Understands issues related to the use of volunteers (training, handling, appropriate use, liability, responsibility).   7.2

Communication/Documentation: Maintains necessary communication and documentation.   8

Understands the chain of communication and role of the PIO.   8.1

Understands basic vocabulary as well as acronyms used in disaster operations.   8.2

Knows basic procedures for medical record-keeping (including data capture and banking, role of toe tags).   8.3

(Contd)

21

Table 1.1b (*Continued*)

	Competency number
Knows basics of evidentiary documentations (crime scene evidence).	8.4
Understands basic types of communications equipment (primary/backup) and the need for and application of basic technical communications security procedures (encryption, varied frequencies).	8.5
Regulatory/Legal/Ethical Principles: Complies with regulatory and legal as well as accepted moral and ethical principles.	9
Understands regulatory and legal landscape as well as moral and ethical issues as they impact on Disaster Medicine. Has sufficient knowledge to operate in compliance with regulatory and ethical principles related to the following: HIPAA, EMTALA/COBRA, Stafford Act, JACHO, Federal Response Plan, OSHA, NIOSH, ADA/Access, Licensing, Sovereign Immunity, Good Samaritan Doctrine, Federal Tort Claims Act, Expectant Patient Issues (dying not yet dead, DNR), NRC, CDC, FDA, EPA, Confidentiality, Consent, Withdrawal of Care, refusal to assume risk, AMA/Refusal of Care, Privacy/Decontamination, profiling, legal rights of responders, professionalism.	9.1
Public Health and Legal Considerations 1–Immediate and Long Range.	9.2
Assessment and Treatment: Assesses and treats injuries resulting from natural/non-natural and incidental/intentional causes in a variety of environments (urban, rural, austere).	10
Has the knowledge and skills to assess and treat injuries related to the following:	10.1
Electrocution – including high voltage/low amperage, high voltage/high amperage, low voltage/high amperage, low voltage/low amperage, AC vs. DC.	10.1.1
Resuscitation Protocols – ACLS, BCLS, PALS, APLS, ALSO, NALS, NRP.	10.1.2
Infection – including bio weapon, epidemic, emerging illness, vaccination needs.	10.1.3
Toxin – including natural vs. synthetic, nerve agents, cholinergic, anticholinergic, biologic, blister agents, enzymatic.	10.1.4
Blast trauma – including physics of explosives; primary, blast trauma affecting gut, lung, ear, eyes; bullets, thermal and radiation burns, secondary blast trauma (smash, spear, gas, glow) and tertiary blast trauma (crush, traumatic or emergency amputation).	10.1.5
Ionizing/Non-Ionizing Radiation – including physics, toxicity, exposure rates and times, iodine prophylaxis, pregnancy risks and treatments/antidotes.	10.1.6
Burns – including thermal, Parkland Formula, BSA burned, chemical, radiation, environmental, special population considerations.	10.1.7

(Contd)

Table 1.1b (Continued)

	Competency number
Psychological/psychiatric trauma	11.2.13
Blunt trauma	11.2.14
Autopsy findings and clinical-pathological correlations	11.3

ACIS, advanced cardiac life support; ADA, Americans with Disabilities Act; ARF, acute renal failure; AMA, American Medical Association; APIS, advanced paediatric life support; ALSO, advanced life support in obstetrics; BCIS, basic cardiac life support; BSA, body surface area; CDC, Centers for Disease Control; CERT, Civilian Emergency Response Teams; DMAT, Disaster Medical Assistance Teams; DMORTs, Disaster Mortuary Operational Response Teams; DNR, do not resuscitate; EPA, Environmental Protection Agency; EMS, Emergency Medical Service; EMTALA, Emergency Medical Treatment and Active labor Act; FBI, Federal Bureau of Investigation; FDA, Food and Drug Administration; FEMA, Federal Emergency Management Association; HEICS, Healthcare Executive Incident Command System; HIPAA, Health Information Portability and Accountability Act; IMSuRTs, International Medical Surgical Response Teams; JCAHO, Joint Commission on the Accreditation of Healthcare Organizations; JumpSTART, Jump Simple Triage and Rapid Transport; LA/COBRA, labor Act/Combined Omnibus Reform Act; MASS, move-assess-sort-send; ME, ?; NAIS, neonatal advanced life support; NDMS, National Disaster Medical System; NGO, Non-Governmental Organizations; NIMS, National Incident Management Systems; NIOSH, National Institute for Occupational Safety and Health; NMRT, National Medical Response Teams; NRC, Nuclear Regulatory Commission; NRF, National Response Framework; NRP, National Response Plan; OSHA, Occupational Safety and Health Administration; PALS, paediatric advanced life support; PPE, personal protective equipment; rxn, reaction; START, simple triage and rapid transport; RPM, respiration pulse mentation; USAMRICD, US Army Medical Research Institute of Chemical Defense; VMAT, Veterinary Medical Assistance Team; WMD-CSTs, weapons of mass destruction-CST.

based on adaptation of Bloom's Cognitive Taxonomy, to allow each health system responder to achieve the highest level of proficiency within each competency. This AMA framework accommodates the development of courses and curricula to meet the diverse education, training, and job requirements of all target groups (see Tables 1.2a and 1.2b).

The key addition of the AMA core competencies is the stratification of the competencies based on the clinical and non-clinical role of the healthcare responder. Basic to the philosophy of both core competency documents is the ideal that all healthcare providers should receive disaster healthcare

Table 1.2a American Medical Association (AMA) Core Competencies for all Health Professionals in a Disaster

Competency domain	Core competencies
1.0 Preparation and Planning	1.1 Demonstrate proficiency in the use of an all-hazards framework for disaster planning and mitigation.
	1.2 Demonstrate proficiency in addressing the health-related needs, values and perspectives of all ages and populations in community and institutional disaster plans.
2.0 Detection and Communication	2.1 Demonstrate proficiency in the detection of and immediate response to a disaster or public health emergency.
	2.2 Demonstrate proficiency in the use of information and communication systems in a disaster or public health emergency.
	2.3 Demonstrate proficiency in addressing cultural, ethnic, religious, linguistic, socioeconomic and special health-related needs of all ages and populations in community and institutional emergency communication systems.
3.0 Incident Management and Support Systems	3.1 Demonstrate proficiency in the initiation, deployment, and coordination of national, regional, state, local and institutional incident command and emergency operations systems.
	3.2 Demonstrate proficiency in the mobilization and coordination of disaster support services.
	3.3 Demonstrate proficiency in the provision of health system surge capacity for the management of mass casualties in a disaster or public health emergency.
4.0 Safety and Security	4.1 Demonstrate proficiency in the prevention and mitigation of health, safety and security risks to yourself and others in a disaster or public health emergency.
	4.2 Demonstrate proficiency in the use of personal protective equipment at a disaster scene or receiving facility.
	4.3 Demonstrate proficiency in victim decontamination at a disaster scene or receiving facility.
5.0 Clinical/Public Health Assessment and Intervention	5.1 Demonstrate proficiency in the use of triage systems in a disaster or public health emergency.

(Contd)

Table 1.2a (*Continued*)

Competency domain	Core competencies
	5.2 Demonstrate proficiency in the clinical assessment and management of injuries, illnesses, and mental health conditions manifested by all ages and populations in a disaster or public health emergency.
	5.3 Demonstrate proficiency in the management of mass fatalities in a disaster or public health emergency.
	5.4 Demonstrate proficiency in public health interventions to protect the health of all ages, populations and communities affected by a disaster or public health emergency.
6.0 Contingency, Continuity and Recovery	6.1 Demonstrate proficiency in the application of contingency interventions for all ages, populations, institutions, and communities affected by a disaster or public health emergency.
	6.2 Demonstrate proficiency in the application of recovery solutions for all ages, populations, institutions and communities affected by a disaster or public health emergency.
7.0 Public Health Law and Ethics	7.1 Demonstrate proficiency in the application of moral and ethical principles and policies for ensuring access to and availability of health services for all ages, populations, and communities affected by a disaster or public health emergency.
	7.2 Demonstrate proficiency in the application of laws and regulations to protect the health and safety of all ages, populations and communities affected by a disaster or public health emergency.

training while those interested in leadership, planning and coordination roles should meet a higher standard.

● Board certification

Physicians who hold board certification in Disaster Medicine have demonstrated by written and simulator-based examination that through training and field experience they have mastered the spectrum of knowledge and skills which defines the

Table 1.2b American Medical Association (AMA) Core and Group-Specific Competencies for Health System Professionals in a Disaster

Competency domains	Core competencies	Category-specific competencies		
		Informed worker/student	Practitioner	Leader
1.0 Preparation and Planning	1.1 Demonstrate proficiency in the use of an all-hazards framework for disaster planning and mitigation.	1.1.1 Describe the all-hazards framework for disaster planning and mitigation. 1.1.2 Explain key components of your regional, community, institutional and personal/family disaster plans.	1.1.3 Summarize your regional, community, office practice and institutional disaster plans. 1.1.4 Perform your expected role in community and institutional disaster exercises and drills. 1.1.5 Conduct hazard vulnerability assessments for your office practice, community or institution.	1.1.6 Participate in the design, implementation and evaluation of disaster exercises and drills to ensure continual assessment of regional, community and institutional disaster plans.
	1.2 Demonstrate proficiency in addressing the health-related needs, values, and perspectives of all ages and populations in community and institutional disaster plans.	1.2.1 Identify individuals (of all ages) and populations with special needs who may be more vulnerable to adverse health effects in a disaster.	1.2.2 Delineate healthcare and public health issues that need to be addressed in community and institutional disaster plans to accommodate the needs, values and perspectives of all ages and populations. 1.2.3 Identify psychological reactions that may be exhibited by victims of all ages, their families and responders in a disaster or public health emergency.	1.2.4 Create, evaluate and revise policies and procedures for meeting the health-related needs of all ages and populations in community and institutional disaster plans.

(Contd)

Table 1.2b (Continued)

Competency domains	Core competencies	Category-specific competencies		
		Informed worker/student	Practitioner	Leader
2.0 Detection and Communication	2.1 Demonstrate proficiency in the detection of and immediate response to a disaster or public health emergency.	2.1.1 Recognize general indicators and epidemiologic clues of a disaster or public health emergency (including natural, unintentional, and terrorist events). 2.1.2 Describe immediate actions and precautions to protect yourself and others from harm in a disaster or public health emergency.	2.1.3 Characterize signs and symptoms, as well as disease and injury patterns, likely to be associated with exposure to natural disasters, conventional and nuclear explosives and/or release of biologic, chemical and radiological agents. 2.1.4 Explain the purpose and role of surveillance systems that can be used to detect and monitor a disaster or public health emergency.	2.1.5 Evaluate and modify policies and procedures for the detection and immediate response to natural disasters, industrial- or transportation-related catastrophes (e.g. hazardous material spill, explosion), epidemics and acts of terrorism (e.g. involving conventional and nuclear explosives and/or release of biologic, chemical and radiological agents).
	2.2 Demonstrate proficiency in the use of information and communication systems in a disaster or public health emergency.	2.2.1 Describe emergency communication and reporting systems and procedures for contacting family members, relatives, coworkers and local authorities in a disaster or public health emergency. 2.2.2 Describe informational resources that are available for health professionals and the public to prepare for, respond to and recover from disasters.	2.2.3 Utilize emergency communications systems to report critical health information to appropriate authorities in a disaster or public health emergency. 2.2.4 Access timely and credible health and safety information for all ages and populations affected by natural disasters, industrial- or transportation-related catastrophes (e.g. hazardous material spill, explosion), epidemics, and acts of terrorism (e.g. involving conventional and nuclear explosives and/or release of biologic, chemical, and	2.2.5 Evaluate and modify risk communication and emergency reporting systems to ensure that health, safety, and security warnings and actions taken, are articulated clearly and appropriately in a disaster or public health emergency.

2.3 Demonstrate proficiency in addressing cultural, ethnic, religious, linguistic, socioeconomic, and special health-related needs of all ages and populations in community and institutional emergency communication systems.

2.3.1 Describe strategies for and barriers to communicating and disseminating health information to all ages and populations affected by a disaster or public health emergency.

2.3.2 Delineate cultural, ethnic, religious, linguistic and health-related issues that need to be addressed in community and institutional emergency communication systems for all ages and populations affected by a disaster or public health emergency.

2.3.3 Create, evaluate and revise policies and procedures for meeting the needs of all ages and populations in community and institutional emergency communication systems.

3.0 Incident Management and Support Systems

3.1 Demonstrate proficiency in the initiation, deployment and coordination of national, regional, state, local and institutional incident command and emergency operations systems.

3.1.1 Describe the purpose and relevance of the National Response Plan, National Incident Management System and Hospital Incident Command System to community and institutional disaster response.

3.1.2 Demonstrate your function and describe other job functions in institutional and community disaster response systems to ensure unified command and scalable response to a disaster or public health emergency.

3.1.3 Devise, evaluate and modify institutional and community incident command and emergency operations systems to ensure unified command and scalable response to a disaster or public health emergency.

(Contd)

Table 1.2b (Continued)

Competency domains	Core competencies	Category-specific competencies		
		Informed worker/student	Practitioner	Leader
	3.2 Demonstrate proficiency in the mobilization and coordination of disaster support services.	3.2.1 Describe global, federal, regional, state, local, institutional, organizational and private industry disaster support services, including the rationale for the integration and coordination of these systems.	3.2.2 Demonstrate the ability to collaborate with relevant public and private sector stakeholders to ensure efficient coordination of civilian, military and other disaster response assets.	3.2.3 Develop, evaluate and revise policies and procedures for mobilizing and integrating global, federal, regional, state, local, institutional, organizational, and private industry disaster support services in a disaster. This includes knowledge of legal statutes and mutual aid agreements for the mobilization and deployment of civilian, military and other response personnel and assets.
	3.3 Demonstrate proficiency in the provision of health system surge capacity for the management of mass casualties in a disaster or public health emergency.	3.3.1 Describe the potential impact of mass casualties on access to and availability of clinical and public health resources in a disaster.	3.3.2 Characterize institutional and community surge capacity assets in the public and private health response sectors and the range of their potential assistance in a disaster or public health emergency.	3.3.3 Develop and evaluate policies, plans, and strategies for predicting and providing surge capacity of institutional and community health systems for the management of mass casualties in a disaster or public health emergency.

4.0 Safety and Security	4.1 Demonstrate proficiency in the prevention and mitigation of health, safety and security risks to yourself and others in a disaster.	4.1.1 Using an all-hazards framework, explain general health, safety and security risks associated with disasters.	4.1.3 Characterize unique health, safety and security risks associated with natural disasters, industrial- or transportation-related catastrophes (e.g. hazardous material spill, explosion), epidemics and acts of terrorism (e.g. involving conventional and nuclear explosives and/or release of biologic, chemical, and radiological agents).	4.1.5 Develop, evaluate, and revise community and institutional policies and procedures to protect the health, safety, and security of all ages and populations affected by a disaster or public health emergency.
		4.1.2 Describe infection control precautions to protect healthcare workers, other responders, and the public from exposure to communicable diseases, such as pandemic influenza.	4.1.4 Utilize federal and institutional guidelines and protocols to prevent the transmission of infectious agents in healthcare and community settings.	
	4.2 Demonstrate proficiency in the use of personal protective equipment at a disaster scene or receiving facility.	4.2.1 Describe the rationale and specific function of personal protective equipment that may be used in a disaster or public health emergency.	4.2.2 Demonstrate the ability to locate and use personal protective equipment according to the degree and type of protection required for various types of exposures.	4.2.3 Develop, evaluate and revise policies, protocols and procedures for the use of all levels of personal protective equipment that may be used at a disaster scene or receiving facility.
	4.3 Demonstrate proficiency in victim decontamination at a disaster scene or receiving facility.	4.3.1 Explain the purpose of victim decontamination in a disaster.	4.3.2 Decontaminate victims at a disaster scene or receiving facility.	4.3.3 Develop, evaluate and revise decontamination policies, protocols and procedures that may be implemented at a disaster scene or receiving facility.

(Contd)

Table 1.2b (Continued)

Competency domains	Core competencies	Category-specific competencies		
		Informed worker/student	Practitioner	Leader
5.0 Clinical/Public Health Assessment and Intervention	5.1 Demonstrate proficiency in the use of triage systems in a disaster or public health emergency.	5.1.1 Explain the role of triage as a basis for prioritizing or rationing healthcare services for victims and communities affected by a disaster or public health emergency.	5.1.2 Explain the strengths and limitations of various triage systems that have been developed for the management of mass casualties at a disaster scene or receiving facility. 5.1.3 Perform mass casualty triage at a disaster scene or receiving facility.	5.1.4 Develop, evaluate and revise mass casualty and population-based triage policies, protocols and procedures that may be implemented in a disaster or public health emergency.
	5.2 Demonstrate proficiency in the clinical assessment and management of injuries, illnesses and mental health conditions manifested by all ages and populations in a disaster or public health emergency.	5.2.1 Describe possible medical and mental health consequences for all ages and populations affected by a disaster or public health emergency. 5.2.2 Explain basic life saving and support principles and procedures that can be utilized at a disaster scene.	5.2.3 Demonstrate the ability to apply and adapt clinical knowledge and skills for the assessment and management of injuries and illnesses in victims of all ages under various exposure scenarios (e.g. natural disasters; industrial- or transportation-related catastrophes; epidemics; and acts of terrorism involving conventional and nuclear explosives and/or release of biological, chemical and radiological agents), in accordance with professional scope of practice. 5.2.4 Identify strategies to manage fear, panic, stress, and other psychological responses that may be elicited by victims, families, and responders in a disaster or	5.2.5 Develop, evaluate and revise policies, protocols and procedures for the clinical care of all ages and populations under crisis conditions, with limited situational awareness and resources.

5.3 Demonstrate proficiency in the management of mass fatalities in a disaster or public health emergency.	5.3.1 Describe psychological, emotional, cultural, religious and forensic considerations for the management of mass fatalities in a disaster or public health emergency.	5.3.2 Explain the implications and specialized support services required for the management of mass fatalities from natural disasters, epidemics and acts of terrorism (e.g. involving conventional and nuclear explosives and/or release of biologic, chemical and radiological agents). 5.3.3 Explain the need for (and the need to collect and preserve) forensic evidence from living and deceased humans and animals at a disaster scene or receiving facility.	5.3.4 Develop, evaluate and revise policies, protocols and procedures for the management of human and animal remains at a disaster scene or receiving facility.
5.4 Demonstrate proficiency in public health interventions to protect the health of all ages, populations and communities affected by a disaster or public health emergency.	5.4.1 Describe short- and long-term public health interventions appropriate for all ages, populations and communities affected by a disaster or public health emergency.	5.4.2 Apply knowledge and skills for the public health management of all ages, populations and communities affected by natural disasters, industrial- or transportation-related catastrophes, epidemics and acts of terrorism, in accordance with professional scope of practice. This includes active/passive surveillance, movement restriction, vector control, mass immunization and prophylaxis, rapid needs assessment, environmental monitoring, safety of food and water, and sanitation.	5.4.3 Develop, evaluate and revise public health policies, protocols and procedures for the management of all ages, populations and communities affected by natural disasters, industrial- or transportation-related catastrophes, epidemics and acts of terrorism.

(Contd)

Table 1.2b (Continued)

Competency domains	Core competencies	Category-specific competencies		
		Informed worker/student	Practitioner	Leader
6.0 Contingency, Continuity and Recovery	6.1 Demonstrate proficiency in the application of contingency interventions for all ages, populations, institutions and communities affected by a disaster or public health emergency.	6.1.1 Describe solutions for ensuring the continuity of supplies and services to meet the medical and mental health needs of yourself, your family, office practice, institution and community in a disaster, under various contingency situations (e.g. mass evacuation, mass sheltering, prolonged shelter-in-place).	6.1.2 Demonstrate creative and flexible decision-making in various contingency situations and risk scenarios, under crisis conditions and with limited situational awareness.	6.1.3 Develop, evaluate and revise contingency and continuity policies and plans for healthcare professionals, institutions and community health systems to maintain the highest possible standards of care under various risk scenarios.
	6.2 Demonstrate proficiency in the application of recovery solutions for all ages, populations, institutions and communities affected by a disaster or public health emergency.	6.2.1 Describe short- and long-term medical and mental health considerations for the recovery of all ages, populations and communities affected by a disaster or public health emergency.	6.2.2 Describe solutions for ensuring the recovery of clinical records, supplies and services to meet the physical and mental health needs of yourself, your family, institution and community in a disaster or public health emergency.	6.2.3 Develop, evaluate and revise policies and plans for the efficient recovery of institutional and community health systems in a disaster or public health emergency.

7.0 Public Health Law and Ethics	7.1 Demonstrate proficiency in the application of moral and ethical principles and policies for ensuring access to and availability of health services for all ages, populations and communities affected by a disaster or public health emergency.	7.1.1 Describe moral and ethical issues relevant to the management of individuals (of all ages), populations and communities affected by a disaster or public health emergency.	7.1.2 Apply moral and ethical principles and policies to address individual and community health needs in a disaster. This includes understanding of professional obligation to treat, the right to protect personal safety in a disaster and responsibilities and rights of health professionals in a disaster or public health emergency.	7.1.3 Develop, evaluate and revise ethical principles, policies and codes to address individual and community health needs in all disaster phases.
	7.2 Demonstrate proficiency in the application of laws and regulations to protect the health and safety of all ages, populations and communities affected by a disaster or public health emergency.	7.2.1 Describe legal and regulatory issues relevant to disasters and public health emergencies, including the basic legal framework for public health.	7.2.2 Apply legal principles, policies and practices to address individual and community health needs in a disaster. This includes understanding of liability, worker protection and compensation, licensure, privacy, quarantine laws and other legal issues to enable and encourage health professionals to participate in disaster response and maintain the highest possible standards of care under extreme conditions.	7.2.3 Develop, evaluate and revise legal principles, policies, practices and codes to address individual and community health needs in all disaster phases

specialty of Disaster Medicine. In the United States of America, this body of knowledge and skills is contained in the core competencies document created and maintained by the ABODM and the AADM. Both the AADM and the ABODM are working with medical organizations and governments around the world to establish Disaster Medicine board certification and training programmes internationally. As with all core competencies documents, the specific knowledge and skills required for certification are subject to constant refinement and evolution. This statement cannot be more true than for a specialty like Disaster Medicine where the nature of the threats faced, the responses undertaken and the lessons learned become more complex with each event.

● Disaster medicine in practice

The practice of Disaster Medicine appears superficially to be sporadic, following the needs created by each disaster. An understanding, however, of the planning, preparation, response and recovery phases associated with the disaster life cycle demonstrates the duality of Disaster Medicine practice. The vast majority of those trained to apply their healthcare skills in austere environments will be sporadic disaster responders; however those 'specializing' in Disaster Medicine will assume roles in the process of healthcare planning and preparation as well as participating in response and recovery leadership. Many ethical, legal and regulatory issues in disaster healthcare are yet to be resolved. Limited resources in light of mass casualties will necessitate decisions that are uncomfortable for healthcare providers accustomed to providing every possible care option to every patient every time. Liability and obligation to provide care provide opposing considerations both legally and ethically. Social responsibility vs. corporate responsibility on the part of private healthcare institutions and hospitals are now ethical, legal and regulatory considerations.

LEARNING POINT

The duality of response stage clinical practice and non-response stage non-clinical practice make Disaster Medicine education necessary for all clinicians and Disaster Medicine certification a must for healthcare leaders.

REFERENCES AND FURTHER READING

References

Barbera JA and McIntyre AG. *Jane's Mass Casualty Handbook: Hospital. Emergency Preparedness and Response*. Jane's Information Group, Ltd, Surrey, UK, 2003.

Marghella P. *National Strategies for Medical Contingency Planning Seminar*. September, 2007.

Ramirez MA. *Symposium on Disaster Preparedness Markets in the United States*. Ft. Lauderdale, FL, September, 2007.

Shultz JM, Espinel Z, Cohen RE, Smith RG, Flynn BW. *Surge, Sort, Support: Disaster Behavioural Health for Healthcare Professionals*. Disaster Life Support Publishing, Inc, Orlando, FL, 2006.

Further reading

Homeland Security Presidential Directives available online from: www.fas.org/irp/offdocs/nspd/index.html

Ramirez MA and Shultz JM. *Surge, Sort, Support Lecture Series*. University of Miami and the Florida Department of Health, 2006.

2 The medical response to domestic terrorism and major incident management

J. P. G. Bolton

● Introduction

The attacks on the World Trade Center in New York in September 2001 and those on the transport systems in Madrid in 2004 and London in July 2005 ushered in a new era of terrorism in the developed world. In these attacks the aim was no-notice indiscriminate attacks on civilian targets. Since then the threat of terrorism has remained high with further failed attacks on aviation targets. This chapter looks at terrorism, possible means of terrorist attack and responses to such attacks. The responses to a terrorist attack are similar to those of any other major disaster and reference is made to other chapters in this book for more information. Where an attack is unconventional such as in the use of chemical, biological, radiological or nuclear agents there will be additional factors to consider such as the limitation of contamination, decontamination, specific treatments and the sequelae of such an attack in terms of long-term health effects.

● Terrorism

Warfare can be categorized as regular or irregular where regular warfare is that fought between the standing military forces of the opposing states. Irregular warfare is practised by participants who are not members of standing armed forces and may involve conflict with regular armed forces such as the French Resistance campaign of the Second World War or the Irish Republican Army (IRA) campaign in the United Kingdom (UK) in the latter part of the twentieth century or fighting between groups of irregular forces such as the warlord conflicts in Darfur and Somalia; the sectarian campaign between the IRA and Loyalist paramilitary groups in Northern Ireland or the Sunni and Shi'a groups in Iraq currently. The UK Ministry of Defence defines irregular activity as:

> 'Behaviour that attempts to effect or prevent change through the illegal use, or threat, of violence conducted by ideologically or criminally motivated non-regular forces, groups or individuals as a challenge to authority.'

Terrorism is a tool of the irregular whose campaigns may be directed against the national administrations, security services, armed forces, economic assets and civilian population of established states. Terrorist incidents seek to terrorize the civilian population and induce the national authorities into responses that cause increasing disruption to the normal business of everyday life and risk becoming intrusively draconian.

Irregular campaigns are almost always long drawn-out affairs such as the Basque separatist and the IRA campaigns of the latter half of the twentieth century in Spain and the UK respectively, both of which ran over decades. Terrorist campaigns in the latter part of the twentieth century, as exemplified above, tended to target military and security forces and economic assets, such as the Canary Wharf and Baltic Exchange attacks by the IRA in London and the Arndale shopping centre in Manchester rather than outrages against the civilian population, although the collateral involvement of civilians did not deter the terrorist as in the pub bombings of the 1970s by the IRA on the UK mainland. The method of attack tended to be the bullet and the bomb but more recently there appears to have been a shift towards targeting the civilian population and the use of other forms of attack, as evidenced by the 1995 Tokyo underground attack, the September 11, 2001 attacks in the USA, the Madrid train and London transport system attacks or the attempted attack on Glasgow airport in June 2007.

● Types of terrorist incident

Terrorist incidents may be overt or covert and this will be determined by the method of attack and the intent of the terrorist. An overt 'big bang attack' will have maximal impact but be of relatively short duration whereas the covert attack using chemical, biological, radiological or nuclear (CBRN) agents may be considerably more disruptive over a longer period of time and cause considerably more 'terror'. Attacks can be classified as follows:

Conventional attack

This type of incident is characterized as conventional because it involves the types of weapons normally associated with warfare, namely the bullet and the bomb or improvised explosive device (IED). It is likely to be an overt rather than a covert attack. The bullet is likely to be a more discriminating form of attack, as in the murder of a member of the security forces, and reduces the chance of adverse publicity by not creating collateral casualties amongst bystanders but the requirement to approach the target and fire a weapon exposes the terrorist to the risk of apprehension or counterattack. The IED is less discriminating but risks causing coincidental casualties amongst the civilian population whose opinion may turn against the terrorists' aims. Its advantage is that it is destructive, can be placed in advance and does not require the terrorist's presence at the scene at the time of detonation.

The mechanisms of wounding are the same as those on the battlefield, namely, **Penetrating, Blunt, Blast and Thermal** and the management of such wounds is discussed in another chapter (see Chapter 8).

Chemical attack

Chemical agents are an attractive proposition to someone wanting to terrorize a civilian community although there are potential problems with achieving remote delivery. They have the advantage that they offer a range of lethality and precision and are potentially able to kill or injure large numbers of people with small amounts of agent compared with the size of bomb required to achieve similar effect. Chemical agents are reasonably easy to produce, requiring neither sophisticated nor bulky equipment and effects can be immediate or delayed and thus the incident can be either an overt or a covert attack. The murder of Georgi Markhov, a Bulgarian dissident who was killed outside the BBC in London in 1978, was ascribed to Eastern bloc agents who used a modified umbrella to inject a small pellet of ricin into his leg. Symptoms of ricin poisoning, which mimicked the prodromal signs and symptoms of an infectious disease, occurred some days after the initial attack thus masking both the time and nature of the assault which went virtually unnoticed by the victim. A more obvious example of a chemical terrorist attack was the unleashing of sarin in the Tokyo underground system in 1995 by the Uhm-Shinrikiu cult which killed 12 people and injured more than 5500. More recently insurgents in Iraq have used industrial chlorine gas disseminated by an explosive device as a method of terrorist attack.

Biological attack

Biological weapons have similar properties as chemical weapons that are of use to the terrorist and indeed the distinction between chemical and biological agents is becoming increasingly blurred as exemplified by ricin. They have a range of lethality and a delayed onset, giving the terrorist the chance to distance himself from the target, and they cause terror. The attack will almost certainly be covert unless the terrorist publicizes the incident and recognition that an attack has occurred may well take time to evolve since the initial phases of any illness caused will almost certainly mimic other less sinister diseases. Indeed if the intent was to cause terror and death it would be an advantage for the agent used to produce signs and symptoms of common infectious diseases rather than something that pointed towards a biological attack as this would delay recognition of the condition and the imposition of control measures. Biological weapons are however difficult to control as was shown by the accidental release of anthrax at the Sverdlovsk biological weapons centre in the USSR in 1979 which resulted in 64 deaths out of 94 infected who were working in a factory downwind of the release, a case fatality rate of 68 per cent. Biological weapons have not been used in modern warfare, but in 2001 anthrax spores were posted to Government offices and media organisations in the aftermath of the September 11 attacks on Washington DC and New York resulting in five deaths from some 22 infected people.

Radiological attack

Radiological attack covers the continuum between nuclear weapons and the use of radiological substances as terror weapons. The world has experienced nuclear attack in the form of the atom bombs dropped on Hiroshima and Nagasaki at the end of the Second World War and the effects, both acute and chronic, are well established. Whilst a nuclear attack may be an unlikely method for a terrorist, the use of radiological substances has greater attraction. In London in 2006, Russian dissident Andrei Litvinenko was killed by being poisoned with polonium 210 at a meeting in a hotel in London. This was a covert attack whose presentation was one of the victims falling acutely ill with no obvious diagnosis being immediately apparent. By the time polonium was implicated some days had passed and there was considerable evidence of contamination of people and property though no further reported illness. The spectre of the 'dirty bomb' namely the dissemination of a radiological substance by an explosive device designed to contaminate large areas and numbers of people is one that receives considerable discussion. The explosion at the Chernobyl nuclear power station in the Ukraine in 1986 was testament, on an altogether larger scale, to the possible effects of such an attack. The local town of Pripiat was evacuated as a result of the explosive spread of radioactive material and remains uninhabitable to this day. That is the spectre of the 'dirty bomb' and the terrorising effects can only be imagined albeit on a smaller scale.

● Emergency service responders to terrorist attack

In the Western democracies terrorism is dealt with under criminal law and thus response to a terrorist incident must include the gathering of evidence alongside the rescue and treatment of the injured. This section will briefly focus on the roles of the major respondents to a terrorist incident and these will be expanded on in subsequent chapters. Table 2.1 lists agencies involved and their role.

Before describing these roles it is worth considering awareness of the threat level. In the UK the Home Office publishes the current security threat level on its website and the Foreign and Commonwealth Office provides similar information about countries overseas.

Police

Apart from any evidence gathering activity, it is only the police who have the authority to direct the public, restrict access, close

PEARL OF WISDOM

In responding to a terrorist incident, as indeed to any other major incident, the police have primacy.

roads, impose cordons and the like. The police take command of an incident and control the activities of other responders. A hierarchical command structure, with representation from all agencies involved, is set up and typically involves a strategic level of command (Gold command in the UK), a tactical command post at the site of the incident but whose responsibility is to take command and control at the scene (Silver command in the UK) and an operational level of command (Bronze command in the UK) which commands those intimately responding to the incident. The police roles are crowd control and marshalling, establishing a cordon, route clearance and traffic control, evacuation, media and public communication operations and in CBRN incidents controlling the clean/dirty areas to prevent the spread of contamination. A major police role is also the establishment of mortuaries and the casualty bureau whereby the dead, injured and missing can be identified and put in contact with relatives.

L **LEARNING POINTS**

Major incidents – command and control

In the United Kingdom there are hierarchical and inter-sectoral command and control arrangements for major incidents known as the Gold, Silver, Bronze system.

Gold Command is the strategic level of command. It concentrates on the strategy for managing an incident. It defines what needs to be done and sets the policy for managing the incident, identifies the resources to be used to respond to the incident and coordinates the responses of the agencies involved. It also determines the most appropriate overall commander, usually police during a response and local authority during recovery, and the relationships with subordinate levels of command. A key task is to establish a multi-sectoral Strategic Coordinating Group.

Silver Command is the tactical level of command and is concerned with how to respond to the incident. It is usually situated outside but close to the incident cordon and manages the incident and the agencies providing on-site resources.

Bronze Command is the operational level of command and is located at the site of the incident. Its concern is the on-site response to the incident with command and control responsibilities for those intimately involved in responding to the incident. Not all levels of the command system will deploy to every incident. One that is small, does not cross administrative boundaries and can be managed by local responders without reinforcement will probably deploy Bronze and Silver commands with Gold command on stand-by. If, however, the incident exceeds the resources of local responders, crosses administrative boundaries or has national or international implications, Gold Command will be stood up to coordinate the higher level activity. Where there is the possibility of Armed Forces involvement it should be noted that the civilian strategic hierarchy of Strategic, Tactical and Operational is different from that of the military in which the tactical level is the lowest and involves the 'doing'.

Fire and rescue services

In the UK the fire service role has progressively included rescue responsibilities as well as traditional firefighting and the Fire and Rescue Act of 2004 mandated the fire services to respond to terrorist incidents. The fire services have similar roles in other developed countries. As a result of traditional fire fighting and rescue duties the fire services are at the forefront of the rescue effort. They have experience in dealing with fires producing complex and toxic chemicals and with chemical spills such as occur in road accidents. They have an extensive range of rescue equipment, are experienced in the use of personal protective equipment

(PPE) and have access to information systems that provide advice on the toxicity of chemicals and their likely spread. In the UK examples are TOXBASE from the National Poisons Information Service and CHEMET from the Meteorological Office which provides information about the likely spread of a chemical plume.

The fire services are also able to deploy decontamination equipment; although this is more readily suited to the decontamination of firefighters wearing PPE, it could be used for the decontamination of large numbers of uninjured or lightly injured victims of an incident. As a general rule in a terrorist incident it will be firefighters who enter the cordon and rescue victims, bringing them to the cordon where they can be handed over to health service responders.

Health services

In the UK, overarching guidance for emergency planning in the health service is produced by the Department of Health, and can be found on their website, from which individual organizations derive their own plans. The obvious on-scene health service response is the ambulance service. Their role is to deploy to the scene and evacuate casualties to an appropriate hospital. Many ambulance services have the ability to deploy a Casualty Clearing Station, an intermediate facility where casualties can receive resuscitation, initial treatment or maintenance in shelter under the supervision of deployed on-site medical teams found from local health care services or providers like the British Association of Immediate Care Specialists (BASICS).

Contamination from a CBRN incident is a major concern and the evacuation of casualties to hospital could easily be a major vector. Ambulance services are developing decontamination facilities for casualties and clearly need a range of monitoring devices to identify contaminated casualties, staff and equipment. It is entirely possible that a proportion of ambulances will be unavailable for evacuation duties because of contamination and

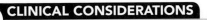

CLINICAL CONSIDERATIONS

An essential role in a major incident involving large numbers of people is the collection and sorting, or triage, of casualties to ensure that those with the greatest need are treated and evacuated first. Most major incident plans involve the sorting of casualties into four categories namely the Dead; Priority 1 who need urgent life and limb saving treatment; Priority 2 whose condition is serious but not immediately life threatening and Priority 3, those who can wait for treatment – the 'walking wounded' in military parlance. Once casualties have been triaged they need to be readily identifiable and the convention is to use a traffic light system of highly visible traffic light coloured cards, bearing clinical details gleaned from the initial triage, to rapidly identify priorities for evacuation (Red for P1, Amber P2 and Green for P3). Triage, of course, is a dynamic process and casualties need to be constantly reassessed for improvement or deterioration in their clinical condition whilst they await evacuation.

may be restricted to the contaminated side of the cordon until they can be cleaned. Hospitals and primary care facilities will have major incident plans which will detail the procedures by which on-site medical teams are despatched to an incident, off-duty staff are called in and beds made available by the early discharge of the less ill patients. In CBRN incidents contamination by casualties poses a considerable threat to the functioning of hospitals and indeed, in the Tokyo subway incident involving the release of a nerve agent, hospital staff were affected by contamination from the casualties. Clear and comprehensive plans are needed to mitigate this risk.

In the UK a further arm of the health service in responding to a terrorist incident is the Health Protection Agency (HPA) and its locally based Health Protection Units. Its role is to provide an integrated approach to protecting UK public health through the

2: The medical response to domestic terrorism and major incident management

provision of support and advice to the NHS, Local Authorities, the emergency services, other arm's length bodies, the Department of Health and devolved administrations and its website provides a wealth of information. Its remit covers infectious diseases and the prevention of harm when hazards involving chemical, poisonous and radiological substances occur. The HPA Centre for Emergency Preparedness provides a central source of authoritative scientific and medical information and other specialist advice on both the planning and operational responses to major incidents and wider public health or other emergencies. In achieving this it provides training courses for the emergency services and coordinates exercises designed to test emergency plans.

Armed forces

As a general rule armed forces have a minimal role in responding to a terrorist incident unless, as in the case of Northern Ireland, they were already deployed in support of the police. Where the armed forces can be of use is in the provision of particular expertise and we are all familiar in the UK with the sight of military bomb or ordnance disposal personnel responding to suspected IEDs. The military is also a source of trained, disciplined

Table 2.1 Agencies which may be involved in major incident command and control and their roles. The following table shows the likely roles of agencies who may be involved in an incident. Depending on their role they may be represented at some or all levels of command. Strategic agencies like government departments would probably only be represented at Gold Command whereas others like the emergency services would probably have representation at all levels.

Police	Overall command and control
	Advice to public
	Communications
	Evacuation
	Protection and preservation of scene
	Investigation of incident
	Casualty information
	Media enquiries

(Contd)

Table 2.1 (*Continued*)

Fire service	Extinguishing fires Rescue Investigation and hazard assessment Identification of chemicals Safety of rescuers Making site safe Decontamination of rescuers, vehicles, walking wounded, and uninjured Clear up
Ambulance services	Evacuation of casualties Decontamination of casualties Medical communications Casualty regulation Provision of on-site treatment facilities
Strategic Health Authorities, Hospitals, Primary Care Trusts	Major incident planning Treatment of casualties Early discharge of hospital patients/alternative hospital/residential accommodation, public information
Health Protection Agency and subordinate Units	Provision of toxicological advice to clinicians, health authorities, emergency services and local authorities Consider evacuation Risk assessment Biological sampling Environmental sampling
Health Protection Agency and subordinate Units	Consideration of follow-up, surveillance and epidemiological studies Public information
Local/Regional authorities	Support emergency services Support community Arrange accommodation for evacuees Coordinate responses of such as utilities, Environment Agency Lead recovery
Utilities	Maintenance of safe services
Health and Safety Executive	Investigate industrial accidents
Department of Trade and Industry/Ministry of Defence	Incidents involving civilian/military nuclear facilities
Food Standards Agency	Potability of food and water
Department of Environment, Transport and Regions	Advice on clearing up, limiting contamination, incidents where transport involved in radiological or chemical spills
Home Office	If sufficiently severe an incident, Home Office would have responsibilities for maintenance of public order, safety and related areas

and organized manpower able to provide a workforce as has frequently been demonstrated in responses to emergency situations like floods around the world. Emergency planners should engage with local military formations to establish what support the military could give in the event of a variety of emergency situations but must fully understand that military forces may not always be available due to other training or operational commitments. In the UK there is a process called Military Aid to the Civil Community which spells out how military forces can be used.

● Responding to a terrorist incident

Conventional attacks

The response to a conventional terrorist incident will be dictated by its scale and the number of casualties that result. As with any violent incident the police will be present and will control access to the scene but the health service response will be as for any small incident involving seriously injured patients. As the size of the incident increases there is a risk that local healthcare facilities will be overwhelmed and major incident plans will be put into action. These are discussed in more detail in other chapters but the principles are that the police cordon off the scene and control access only permitting this when it is safe to do so; the fire service enters the cordon with specialized rescue equipment if required and bring out casualties to a point where they can be handed over to the ambulance service. The ambulance service establishes a presence at each level of command, evacuates casualties to hospital, regulates casualty flow and establishes communications with receiving hospitals and may well set up a casualty clearing station on site. Receiving hospitals initiate their major incident plans, freeing up beds by the early discharge of patients and calling in staff to manage the extra patients and they may despatch site medical teams if there is a requirement.

The London Bombings 7 JULY 2005 (HMSO, 2006)

- 08.50 Explosions on Underground trains at Aldgate, Edgware Road and Russell Square.
- 09.15 Commenced evacuating entire London Underground network.
- 09.50 Explosion on bus at Tavistock Square.
- 56 dead, more than 700 injured.
- London Fire Brigade deployed 240 firefighters, 42 front-line appliances and nine Fire Rescue Units out of a total of 196 vehicles available in London.
- London Ambulance Service deployed more than 200 vehicles and over 400 staff.
- All injured were rescued, medically assessed, treated and, if necessary evacuated to hospital within 3 hours.
- All London hospitals were placed on major incident alert and rapidly made 1200 beds available under major incident plans.
- Of the 700 injured, 103 were admitted to hospital, including 21 critically injured.
- Metropolitan Police Gold Commander held the first meeting of the emergency services Gold Coordinating Group at 10.00 hours.
- Central Government crisis management arrangements activated with the first meeting of Ministers and officials in the Government's crisis management centre held at 10.00 hours.

Overt chemical or radiological attacks

An overt attack involving chemical or radiological agents presents a different situation. The scale of such attacks will be larger; the Tokyo sarin attacks caused casualties numbering in the thousands. Once the use of such materials is recognized, rescuers will be forced to wear protective clothing with consequent restrictions on their ability to communicate with one another and the casualties and severe limitations on the workload they can endure without themselves suffering degradation.

⚡ **HAZARD**

Decontamination poses a major problem. Whilst the fire services have decontamination equipment and a role in decontaminating casualties, this utilizes the same equipment as is used to decontaminate firefighters dressed in PPE and may not be appropriate for seriously injured casualties. Ambulance services are developing decontamination capabilities for such casualties. Limitation of contamination is another problem that requires strict enforcement of cordons and identification of clean and dirty (or contaminated) areas.

There is a risk that equipment and vehicles and even hospitals become contaminated as shown in the Tokyo sarin attack. Limiting contamination is a major and difficult problem and not one that can be easily solved in response to an incident. Clear plans for managing contaminated casualties need to be drawn up and exercised prior to the event, and redundancy needs to be built in since it is almost inevitable that some contaminated casualties will have been evacuated before the nature of the problem has become clear. Once the causative agent has been identified there may be specific treatments. Nerve agent poisoning generally responds to the administration of atropine, oximes and anticonvulsants but the agents are highly toxic and large numbers of patients may need prolonged respiratory support, and these are just the facilities that will not be freed up by the early discharge of existing hospital patients so patients will have to be dispersed. Equally, hospitals may not hold large amounts of antidotes and national stockpiles will have to be released and distributed. In the UK, the HPA maintains the national stockpile and arranges for its release.

CLINICAL CONSIDERATIONS

Nerve agent poisoning (Tokuda *et al.*, 2006)

Physical features: Colourless, tasteless usually odourless liquids which usually evaporate at much the same rate as water.

Routes of absorption: Inhalation, contact with skin and mucous membranes, crossing the cornea particularly easily, and ingestion.

Symptoms: Those of cholinergic overload affecting peripheral and central nervous systems. Muscarinic signs and symptoms are: blurred vision, rhinorrhoea, headache, hypersecretion of lachrymal, salivary, sweat and bronchial glands, cramp-like abdominal pain, miosis, nausea, vomiting, diarrhoea, faecal and urinary incontinence and dyspnoea. Nicotinic effects: skeletal muscle twitching and cramping followed by weakness and flaccid paralysis, tachycardia and hypertension. Central nervous system signs and symptoms are irritability, ataxia, seizures and respiratory depression. Death occurs after convulsions and respiratory failure.

Treatment: Responders must wear appropriate protective clothing to prevent contamination. Casualties must be decontaminated. General supportive measures, especially respiratory support. Specific treatment: Atropine in 2 mg increments to combat the muscarinic effects, repeated every 5–10 minutes, until breathing and secretions improve. There is no upper limit to the dose required but the severely poisoned adult may require 20–30 mg. Pralidoxime chloride reactivates acetylcholinesterase, the enzyme inhibited by nerve agents and organophosphorus insecticides, but must be given before the agent ages whereby it forms an irreversible bond with the enzyme thus preventing its reactivation. A maximum dose of 1800 mg per hour is recommended to prevent excessive blood pressure elevation. In hospital with appropriate monitoring this dose can be exceeded to a maximum of 2500 mg given intravenously over 1–1.5 hours and this may succeed in reactivating more cholinesterase. Diazepam is used to control convulsions and patients may require 30–40 mg intramuscularly. Specific treatment and general supportive measures may need to be continued for some hours or even days whilst the cholinesterase system is reactivated.

Covert attacks

Almost without exception these will be chemical, biological, radiological or nuclear attacks and a key problem will be the recognition that such an attack has occurred. It is likely that the first indications will come from a patient presenting for treatment with an atypical presentation of illness, as in the cases of Georgi Markhov and Alexander Litvinenko suffering from ricin and polonium poisoning respectively, or from requests for assistance with a number of people who have 'collapsed'. UK ambulance services are trained to approach such incidents with great caution in case there has been a chemical release. Krivoy and colleagues (2005), feel that it is essential to determine if there has been a chemical release and if so whether it is an organo-phosphate (OP) compound such as a nerve agent because of the availability of specific antidotes which are most beneficial given early. They propose the following algorithm as a scheme for managing chemical incidents (Fig. 2.1).

In the Markov case there was just a single patient but in the Litvinenko case, Rubin and colleagues (2007) reported that a further 117 people were concerned that their health might have been affected by exposure to polonium and in both cases some days had elapsed between initial presentation and identification of the cause of the illness whereby corrective action could be taken. Clinical and laboratory staff are firmly

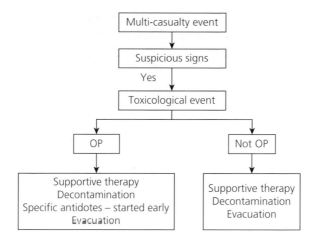

Fig. 2.1 Algorithm for chemical incident management. OP, operational.

in the front line in determining whether there has been such an attack and must constantly be alert to the possibility of malicious attack when faced with atypical illness, but must also be alert to the possibility that an outbreak of communicable disease was caused by deliberate contamination of, say, a water supply. Consider the US anthrax attacks which occurred soon after the World Trade Center attacks and ask yourself how quickly they might have been recognized had they not occurred in such close time proximity to that incident. Detection of such attacks will be as a result of recognition that there is something atypical going on and subsequent high quality traditional epidemiological outbreak investigation aimed at defining who was affected where and when and identifying further contacts. Treatment and outbreak control measures will depend on the cause of the incident but investigation will also be responsible for gathering the evidence with which to find and prosecute the perpetrators.

● Sequelae

As mentioned above, terrorism is dealt with under the criminal law and one obvious consequence of an attack is the police investigation but what about the victims of an attack, both those injured and not? There is intense discussion in the mass media of the psychological effects of a major disaster. Post-traumatic stress disorder (PTSD) is increasingly expected as the result of severe or life-threatening events and the literature is vast. Estimating the extent is difficult but a number of studies provide the following examples of prevalence. Overall lifetime prevalence of PTSD in the US population is reported by Keane and colleagues (2006) to be 7–9 per cent, but in victims of trauma this may be as much as 25–30 per cent (Grinage, 2005). A prevalence study of PTSD, reported by Perrin and co-workers (2007), in those responding to the World Trade Center attacks of 2001, revealed an overall prevalence among rescue/recovery workers of 12.4 per cent ranging from 6.2 per cent in police to 21.2 per cent in unaffiliated helpers with the risks being greater in those who performed tasks not common to their occupation. The suggestion that cohesion and training may be protective is suggested by the finding by the King's College, London, Military Health Research Unit (2006), that the prevalence of PTSD among UK military personnel who participated in the Iraq war of 2003 was around 4 per cent. Amongst victims of a terrorist incident the prevalence of PTSD, the most common psychological condition, may well be in the region of 35 per cent (Conejo-Galindo *et al.*, 2007). To prevent PTSD occurring, single-session psychological debriefing was routinely recommended in response to traumatic incidents, but Bisson (2003) has subsequently doubted its efficacy and its routine use is now no longer recommended.

PEARL OF WISDOM

Recognition that post-traumatic stress disorder may arise in victims and responders is necessary and services need to be provided to respond to this need.

While a conventional attack may produce physical and psychological disability amongst those involved, CBRN incidents may well produce 'mystery illness' consequences that the media will highlight and which will require extensive epidemiological investigation. Following the 1991 Gulf Conflict, stories of a mysterious 'Gulf War Syndrome' affecting mainly US and UK veterans began to emerge. Immunizations, medical countermeasures, pesticides, depleted uranium, sand particles, and low concentration nerve agent exposures were among many possible exposures that were implicated. Ultimately large amounts of money were spent on research but despite intensive epidemiological, clinical and basic scientific investigation no convincing evidence of a unique Gulf War related illness ever emerged. Similarly following an air accident in 1992 in Amsterdam where an Israeli cargo plane allegedly carrying a hazardous cargo, reports of ill-health among survivors and rescuers also emerged culminating in further requirements for research into a mystery illness. An epidemiological study was undertaken by Slottje and colleagues (2005 a,b) and has produced a number of publications which have shown that, while exposed workers complained more of symptoms of autoimmune conditions compared with similar control groups, there were no differences in a number of clinical markers of autoimmune disease. There have been suggestions of similar unexpected illnesses following the Tokyo sarin attacks and in those who have had occupational exposures to sheep dips.

A paper by Boin and colleagues in 2001 discusses the emergence of a **'toxic fear'** following such events and recommends a robust risk communications strategy and attention to the long-term sequelae of such incidents rather than achieving rapid closure of an incident. The study into the public information needs following the Litvinenko poisoning found that 11.7 per cent of the study sample perceived that their health was at risk and felt that this proportion was low given that radiation was involved. The reason for this low level of concern was put down to the success of the HPA risk communication effort and individual perceptions that they were not the targets of the attack. The study concluded that it was important to provide the public with detailed, comprehensive information in such circumstances.

There is no reason to suppose that such a risk communication campaign following a terrorist attack would be any less successful.

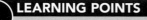

LEARNING POINTS

- Terrorist incidents may be conventional or involve the use of C, B, R or N agents and these may be overt or covert attacks.
- Police have primacy in the response to a terrorist incident and along with saving life and preventing damage to infrastructure the gathering of evidence is an important activity.
- The management of a major terrorist incident is essentially the same as for any other major incident.
- The management of casualties from a conventional terrorist attack will be similar to the management of battle casualties and will follow the principles of military surgery.
- C, B, R or N incidents pose different problems:
    - Recognition that an attack has occurred may be difficult. Clinical staff need to be alert to the possibility when there are unusual cases or patterns of illness.
    - The control of spread of contamination is a huge problem.
    - Decontamination of casualties is vital but may delay access to medical care.
    - Major incident plans need to consider the problems of large numbers of contaminated casualties.
    - There may be specific antidotes but there may also be limited stockpiles.
- Apart from the physical injuries, there may be psychological consequences from the now well-recognized PTSD to the less obvious health concerns arising from potential exposures to toxic chemicals, radiation or biological agents – the concept of toxic fear.
- A good risk communication strategy will help with this aspect.

Summary

Terrorism attempts to effect or prevent change through the illegal use, or threat, of violence conducted by ideologically or criminally motivated non-regular forces, groups or individuals as a challenge to authority. Its nature has changed over recent years with unannounced attacks aimed at the civilian community becoming more common. Most attacks are conventional but the threat of CBRN incidents is increasing and in Western democracies the threat of terrorist attack remains high. Police have primacy in managing a terrorist incident and fire and health services work very much as they do in a major incident. The HPA has a significant role in preparing emergency services for an unconventional terrorist incident. The role of armed forces tends to be small and to concentrate on areas of particular expertise. Responses to a terrorist incident will be as for any major incident save that, if CBRN agents are involved, the threat of contamination, the need to decontaminate victims and the requirement for responders to wear PPE will severely hamper rescue operations. Apart from the physical consequences of an attack, there will be psychological consequences, mainly PTSD, among victims and responders. An unconventional incident may well give rise to a 'toxic fear' or 'mystery illness' which may well involve expensive and extensive research to unravel. There is evidence that in these circumstances a risk communication strategy that is both comprehensive and comprehensible will reduce these unexpected sequelae of an incident.

REFERENCES AND FURTHER READING

References

Bisson JI. Single session early psychological interventions following traumatic events. *Clinical Psychological Review* 2003; **23** (3): 481–99.

Boin A, Van Duin M and Heyse L. Toxic fear: the management of uncertainty in the wake of the Amsterdam air crash. *Journal of Hazardous Materials* 2001; **88** (2–3): 213–34.

Conejo-Galindo J, Medina O, Fraguas D *et al.* Psychopathological sequelae of the 11 March terrorist attacks in Madrid: an epidemiological study of victims treated in a hospital. *European Archives of Psychiatry and Clinical Neurosciences* 2007; **258** (1): 28–34.

Grinage BD. Diagnosis and management of post-traumatic stress disorder. *American Family Physician* 2003; **68** (12): 2401–09.

HMSO. *Addressing Lessons from the Emergency Response to the 7 July 2005 London Bombings: What we learned and what we are doing about it.* 22 September 2006.

Hotopf M, Hull L, Fear N *et al.* The health of UK military personnel who deployed to the 2003 Iraq war: a cohort study. *Lancet* 2006; **367**: 1731–41.

Keane TM, Marshall AD and Taft CT. Posttraumatic stress disorder: etiology, epidemiology and treatment outcome. *Annual Review of Clinical Psychology* 2006; **2**: 161–97.

Krivoy A, Laysih I, Rotman E *et al.* OP or not OP: the medical challenge at the chemical terrorism scene. *Prehospital and Disaster Medicine* 2005; **20**(3): 155–58.

Perrin MA, DiGrande L, Wheeler K *et al.* Differences in PTSD prevalence and associated risk factors among World Trade Center disaster rescue and recovery workers. *American Journal of Psychiatry* 2007; **164**(9): 1385–94.

Rubin GJ, Page L, Morgan O *et al.* Public information needs after the poisoning of Alexander Litvinenko with polonium-210 in London: cross sectional telephone survey and qualitative analysis. *British Medical Journal* 2007; **335**: 1143–6.

Slottje P, Bijisma JA, Smidt N *et al.* Epidemiologic study of the autoimmune health effects of a cargo aircraft disaster. *Archives of Internal Medicine* 2005a; **165**(19): 2280–85.

Slottje P, Huizink AC, Twisk JW *et al.* Epidemiological study air disaster in Amsterdam (ESADA): study design. *BMC Public Health* 2005b; **5**(1): 54.

Tokuda Y, Kikuchi M, Takahashi O and Stein GH. Prehospital management of sarin nerve gas terrorism in urban settings: 10 years of progress after the Tokyo subway sarin attack. *Resuscitation* 2006; **68**: 193–202.

Further reading

Threat levels and advice: www.homeoffice.gov.uk/security/current-threat-level/ and for overseas advice www.fco.gov.uk/servlet/Front?pagename=OpenMarket/Xcelerate/ShowPage&c=Page&cid=1007029390590

Emergency planning:
- Emergency Preparedness www.ukresilience.info/
- UK Government Emergency Planning Training website www.epcollege.gov.uk/
- Department of Health Emergency Planning Policy and Guidance www.dh.gov.uk/en/Policyandguidance/Emergencyplanning/index.htm
- Health Protection Agency: www.hpa.org.uk/

Local Health Authority, Primary Care Trust, Hospital Trust, Local Authority Emergency Plans will be tailored to the local situation and will give the local approach to major incident.

3 Managing national mass casualty incidents

Pietro D. Marghella

'The noise of the fourteen thousand aeroplanes advancing in open order… but in the Kurfurstendamnn and the Eighth Arrondissement, the explosion of anthrax bombs is hardly louder than the popping of a paper bag.' Aldous Huxley, *Brave New World* (1932)

● Introduction

A critic of Aldous Huxley once noted with the smug certainty of a contemporary that 'one vast and obvious failure of foresight is immediately apparent (in that) *Brave New World* contains no reference to nuclear fission.' It is interesting to note, however, that Huxley's prognostications in 1932 *did* foresee the use of biological weapons. Perhaps he was far more visionary than anyone has given him credit for. With the demise of the Soviet Union – the United States' former malefactor-partner in the concept of mutually assured destruction – the threat of nuclear Armageddon virtually has been eliminated, but as many of the leading minds of science, politics, and the military have said, (at least one of) the new 'threat(s) du jour' is the weaponized bio-agent. Perhaps we have come full circle, back to Huxley's predictions of the future world.

The reality of events some 60 years after Huxley's famous work of fiction – one that portended tectonic shifts in the world order – makes Dr. Lederberg's words even more profound, as they speak of a massive paradigm shift regarding threat and international security. For time immemorial, warfare has been largely *linear* and *symmetrical;* that is, large force-on-force engagements with traditional weapons systems have dominated the battlespace. The economic super-engines capable of generating the bigger, better, faster military forces stood to win the battle flags and carry the day as the regional, if not the global, hegemonic powers. Unless a potential challenger to those powers possessed sufficient economic resources to muster adequate force-on-force capabilities, they were largely forced to play a lesser role on the global stage and accept the changing tides of history as their *fait accompli.*

A watershed event in 1983 changed all of that. The terrorist bombing of the US Marine Corps Barracks in Beirut can be seen as the opening gambit in a new era of warfare, when ideological and/or religious enemies of global hegemonic powers first grasped that they could achieve their 'security' objectives quite handily using non-traditional weapons systems and tactics, without the need to engage in force-on-force tactics which would lessen their advantage. With a seemingly synchronized march forward of attacks around the world at a set periodicity of one attack at almost every 2.5 years, the Al Qaeda network – the most obvious and apparently dedicated terrorist organization in the world – successfully executed the worst attack on U.S. soil in the Nation's history with the 9/11 attacks on New York and Washington, DC. At the dawn of the new millennium, the events of 9/11 and the subsequent bombings in Madrid and London have demonstrated that the 'battlefield' is no longer a distant place and that these strategic-impact acts of terrorism have ushered us into the **'Era of Asymmetrical Threats'**.

THINKING POINT

It is now entirely reasonable to expect that there may be future events involving chemical, biological, radiological, nuclear or high-explosive agents with the inherent potential to cause catastrophic levels of casualties, as terrorist organizations seek to continue their campaign against their US and European enemies.

The 2004 Tsunami in Southeast Asia; the 2005 earthquake in Pakistan and hurricanes in the United States Gulf Region; the 2008 earthquake in China; and, most recently, the 2010 earthquake that devastated the impoverished nation of Haiti have demonstrated that natural disasters have as much (or more) potential for death, injury, and/or destruction of critical infrastructure as any man-made threats. All of these hazards (natural or man-made) have the potential to produce a series of cascading effects that make effective response and recovery difficult or, in some cases, impossible.

In the wake of these repeated terrorist attacks and devastating natural disasters, in 2009–10 we were faced with an outbreak of a novel human influenza that reached pandemic proportion with lightening rapidity. Scientists have long warned that we are well overdue for a strain of flu that could far outstrip the last great influenza outbreak, the 1918–19 pandemic which is believed to have caused almost 100 million deaths worldwide. While this most recent pandemic thankfully never achieved anything near such a deadly impact as its predecessor event, its sudden presentation demonstrates that we continue to live in an era beset by threats, and that we will continue to face Herculean challenges in trying to conduct incident management against scenarios that are by their very nature overwhelming.

PEARL OF WISDOM

'The single biggest threat to man's continued dominance on the planet is the virus.' Joshua Lederberg, PhD, Nobel Laureate

The purpose of this chapter is to describe the role of the medical and public health community in preparing for and responding to national mass casualty incidents, and to discuss a number of theories in catastrophic casualty event incident management.

For the purposes of this discussion, the reader is asked to consider two key operative assumptions:

> **THINKING POINTS**
>
> 1. Among the universally accepted critical infrastructure and key resource (CI/KR) sectors (i.e. banking and finance; chemical; commercial facilities; commercial nuclear reactors, materials, and waste; dams; defense industrial base; drinking water and wastewater treatment systems; emergency services; energy; food and agriculture; government facilities; information technology; national monuments and icons; postal and shipping; public health and healthcare; telecommunications; and transportation systems), public health and healthcare is pre-eminent since this sector most directly impacts on the health, safety and survivability of populations affected by disasters.
> 2. It logically follows that if the public health and healthcare sectors fail to prepare for national mass casualty events, it is reasonable to expect catastrophic failures in those CI/KR sectors and an attendant collapse in the ability to adequately execute an incident management mission.

● Defining the spectrum of threat

The US Department of Defense defines a mass casualty incident as:

> 'Any large number of casualties produced in a relatively short period of time, usually as the result of a single incident such as a military aircraft accident, hurricane, flood, earthquake or armed attack that exceeds local logistic support capabilities.'

While it is technically true that as little as three critical care victims of an automobile accident presenting to an under-staffed and ill-equipped hospital emergency room can qualify as a 'mass casualty incident', for the purposes of this chapter we are going to refine our discussion to mass casualty events that can be defined as 'Incidents of National Significance'.

Incidents of National Significance are high impact events that require an extensive and well-coordinated multi-agency response to save lives, reduce damage, and provide the basis for long-term community and economic recovery. Incidents of National Significance fall into seven categorical or 'typed' areas:

- biological incident (natural or terrorist-induced)
- catastrophic incident
- cyber incident
- food and agriculture incident
- nuclear/radiological incident
- oil or hazardous material incident
- terrorist incident.

In 2004, at the direction of the White House's Homeland Security Council, the US Department of Homeland Security created the National Planning Scenarios (NPS), which attempt to articulate the full spectrum of hazards that exist as omnipresent threat (natural and man-made) in today's environment.

Scenario 1:   Nuclear detonation – 10-kiloton improvised nuclear device.
Scenario 2:   Biological attack – aerosol anthrax.
Scenario 3:   Biological disease outbreak – pandemic influenza.
Scenario 4:   Biological attack – plague.
Scenario 5:   Chemical attack – blister agent.
Scenario 6:   Chemical attack – toxic industrial chemicals.
Scenario 7:   Chemical attack – nerve agent.
Scenario 8:   Chemical attack – chlorine tank explosion.
Scenario 9:   Natural disaster – major earthquake.
Scenario 10: Natural disaster – major hurricane.
Scenario 11: Radiological attack – radiological dispersal devices.

Scenario 12: Explosives attack – bombing using improvised explosive devices.

Scenario 13: Biological attack – food contamination.

Scenario 14: Biological attack – foreign animal disease (foot and mouth disease).

Scenario 15: Cyber attack.

The NPS provide more granular theoretical, but highly plausible, illustrative planning scenarios on what Incidents of National Significance may look like and help to define the preparedness requirements that will be needed to effectively prosecute these high-impact events. It is important to note that the NPS contain threat scenarios that are geographically endemic to the United States. Any national-specific planning and preparedness initiatives that choose to replicate this highly useful initiative should carefully consider what specific threats are endemic to their geographic location when attempting to articulate the spectrum of threat.

● Defining the spectrum of response

Figure 3.1 presents the classic operational continuum of a disaster from a horizontal perspective. As the event magnitude increases in scope and scale, we see an associated increase in the event capacity for casualty production on the y axis as well as an increase for the response requirement along the x axis moving from the tactical (local, i.e. city and county) response through the operational (i.e. state and regional) response and finally the strategic (i.e. national). Note that it is theoretically possible to predict the response times associated with each 'frame' of response requirement and that these can be used as planning factors when developing incident management plans within each 'silo' of response. Note, as well, that the slide depicts the location of the historical command and control (C^2) breakpoints along the operational continuum, where fractures predictably occur due to a lack of commonality in the approaches to planning and response secondary to dissimilar perspectives and a lack of collaboration.

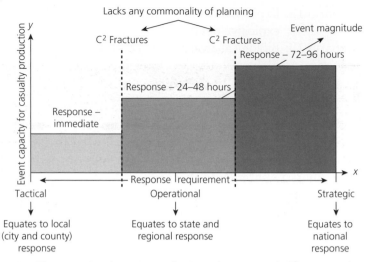

Fig. 3.1 The operational continuum (horizontal perspective). C^2, command and control.

Figure 3.2 is a similar presentation on the operational continuum seen from the vertical perspective. The thin left arrow demonstrates that requirements increase as the size and scope of the event increases, while the thin right arrow demonstrates that capabilities will decrease in loci most proximal to the event as the event expansion occurs. When this happens, it is reasonable to expect that national incident management response involvement will have to occur since those levels of authority would at least theoretically have control of national response assets. The significant delay that is always associated with the national level of response in the operational continuum, however, can and will have a significant deleterious effect on the impacted population. Therefore, as the large arrow on the left demonstrates, if you enhance the most localized response assets at the tactical and microtactical levels (e.g. individual hospitals) and follow preparedness initiatives to support these levels at one layer in the operational continuum to the low operational level (i.e. county response), you effect a 'bottom up' preparedness and response capability

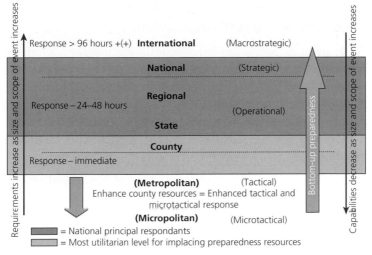

Fig. 3.2 The operational continuum (vertical perspective).

that supports the axiom of 'leadership is local' in a disaster and begins our argument for adequately building surge capacity for national mass casualty incidents.

● Surge capacity planning
Background

With the creation of the 'Catastrophic Incident Response Plan' (which now exists as the Catastrophic Incident Annex in the current US National Response Framework), planners identified seven categorical areas in the public health and healthcare sector that must be addressed in any preparedness and response planning initiative related to national mass casualty incidents. They are:

- surge capacity planning
- patient movement and transportation
- medical logistics and supply
- mass fatality management
- psychosocial support to affected populations

- public health and healthcare crisis communications
- managing special needs populations.

These areas of focus are conspicuously important when any high-end scenario is addressed and it should be noted that they are largely confluent to one another in execution. However, for the purposes of this chapter, we are going to focus on the issue of surge capacity planning and its role of pre-eminent importance in planning for an adequate public health and healthcare response.

Since 9/11 we have seen the emergence of homeland security initiatives around the world that have focused heavily on preventing terrorist attacks (i.e. the 'detect to deter' and 'detect to defend' missions) and (to a lesser extent) on managing the consequences of an attack or a large scale natural disaster. **One area that has universally received far too little attention is our medical infrastructure.** In 2008 congressional hearings in the United States pointed out that this is the one area that potentially represents our greatest single vulnerability at this time. For the purposes of this discussion consider the following: the results of the attacks on New York and Washington, DC in 2001 were catastrophic by any definition. However, it should be carefully pointed out that in both cases there were more fatalities than casualties requiring critical care support. This has been referred to as a 'catastrophic casualty anomaly'. Had the reverse been true, it is questionable whether regional medical capabilities going out several hundred miles distally from New York City could have absorbed the casualty load.

In advance of our discussion on models and theoretical approaches to managing surge in an event of national significance, it is important to note that in a crisis the focus will shift from individual-based care to population-based outcomes. Rather than asking whether or not an individual can be saved, medical professionals will be forced to shift to a 'for the greater good' model and assess how many other people

CASE STUDY

The Madrid rail bombing

The case study for what really would occur in a national mass casualty incident happened on March 11, 2004, when terrorists bombed the rail stations in downtown Madrid. With a casualty load of just under 2000 victims requiring critical care support for poly-trauma, the modern, highly westernized healthcare infrastructure of the entire city was adjudicated as being overwhelmed within hours of the attacks. This is the reality of why surge capacity planning is so important for anything related to a national mass casualty incident. The fact is, even for developed nations, in the event of a terrorist attack or a natural disaster with thousands of persons needing medical attention, there will be insufficient resources to support the affected population if pre-event deliberate planning has not been done to address surge. The ability of our public health and healthcare system to respond to catastrophic events and save as many lives as possible will remain the single most important measure of national preparedness.

would be put at risk if they take the time to save the one, when the goal is to save the many.

● The behavioural model of surge

The typical model of healthcare surge is based on the statistical analysis of past hazard events to create actuarial projections of casualties and fatalities for future hazards relative to a standardized hazard vulnerability. The data collected historically centre on four large groups:

- those with documented physical injury
- those with documented symptoms of physical injury in the absence of physical injury (psychogenic illness)

- those with documented traumatic stress-related illness
- event-related fatalities.

This grouping of data introduces a prejudice that results in a significant underestimation of the size of the potential surge on civilian healthcare institutions. The models also ignore ethical, moral and legal obligations created to guide the behaviour of individual healthcare providers and healthcare institutions in the treatment of individual patients during non-crisis operations. Unfortunately, these ethical, moral and legal considerations have no currently accepted exemptions for crisis or disaster operations.

The wave

A behavioural model of surge is based on a deconstruction of the historical data for disasters. First enunciated by Shultz *et al.* (2003, 2006), the behavioural model builds on the concept of 'upside down triage' (Davis, 2004) and assumes that formal Emergency Medical Service (EMS) transported patients represent the smallest percentage of the total healthcare surge in a mass casualty event. In his review of the historical data since 1978, Shultz found that each EMS patient represented four patients who arrived to the healthcare facility by a means other than EMS transport.

These 'self-transported' patients were typically less severely injured than the EMS patients but arrived to the healthcare facility before the EMS transported patients, thus representing an opportunity for the ill-prepared facility to become overloaded before the critical patients arrived. The EMS and 'self-transported' patients together represent the total number of physically injured patients typically counted in other surge models.

The surge

In addition to these patients, Shultz identified from the historical data patients with physical symptoms clearly of psychogenic origin, i.e. patients with no physical injury on examination and later follow-up. These patients have been typically classified as either 'Mass Psychogenic Illness' (MPI) or 'Multiple Unexplained Physical Symptoms' (MUPS) although the field term 'Walking Wounded' has come into common, if inappropriate, usage. As with the 'self-transported' patients, patients with psychogenic illness present in a minimum ratio of 4 to 1 compared with the total patients with physical injuries, or a 25 to 1 ratio compared with the EMS transported patients.

● The tsunami

The behavioural model first met the legal constraints of medical practice when Shultz and Ramirez (2007) examined the friends and bystanders arriving to the hospital or healthcare facility with the physical and psychological injury patients. Although there is much statistical variation, there is no doubt that the minimum ratio of these 'co-arrivals' is 1 to 1 compared with the total of physical and psychological patients, i.e. this doubles the surge. Under ordinary daily operations, these 'co-arrivals' would not be considered patients under any legal definition and thus would not be part of a 'surge'. However, in the initial hours of a mass casualty response, the hospital or healthcare facility should be under 'limited secure access' and possibly even 'decontamination for access' operations. This creates the need for the 'co-arrivals' to request an evaluation prior to entry into the facility. This evaluation necessarily includes one or more billable medical procedures to occur after the 'co-arrival' crosses the hospital's property line. When any individual requests a billable medical procedure (including a basic evaluation for contamination or decontamination) after crossing the hospital's property line, that individual is legally a patient under the US 1986 Emergency Medical Treatment and Active Labor Act (EMTALA) and its subsequent amendments. Thus the patient surge has risen to a 50 to 1 ratio when compared with EMS transported patients.

This same consideration is applied to the additional groups more recently identified as contributing to the behavioural surge model. The 2004 bombing of trains in Madrid, Spain gave an insight into the behaviour of the largest portion of a healthcare surge, those searching for missing loved ones. The Madrid experience found that for each person already at the hospital as a result of the bombing (patients and family), there would arrive at least one person searching for a loved one NOT at the particular hospital. This 1 to 1 ratio of searching citizens to patients and family resulted in an effective doubling of the surge at every hospital that received patients from the attack. Initially thought to be an anomaly, the same ratios were seen following the collapse of the Interstate 35 West Bridge in Minneapolis, Minnesota.

Unlike the physical injury patient surge, psychological injury and the more massive 'co-arrival' and 'searching citizen' surge components are unchanged in mass fatality events. At best the mass fatality event may represent a 5% reduction in surge based on all physically injured patients dying.

THINKING POINT

Historically, the 100 to 1 surge to Emergency Medical Services ratio of mass casualty events approximates to the 100 to 1 surge to fatally injured ratio seen in mass fatality events.

● Best practice guidance

PEARL OF WISDOM

'I'd rather prepare our citizens than mourn them.'
President Ronald Reagan

In 2004, the US Department of Health and Human Services – the Federal Partner Agency assigned national responsibility for Emergency Support Function #8 (Public Health and Medical Services) under the National Response Framework – issued benchmark guidance on the medical management of large-scale disasters, entitled *Medical Surge Capacity and Capability* (CNA, 2004).

The premise of this national surge capacity planning initiative is consistent with the points previously mentioned in this chapter. Public health and healthcare systems must prepare for major emergencies or disasters, as the common denominator to any of these events will be human casualties. It should be assumed that such events will severely challenge the ability of healthcare systems to adequately care for large numbers of patients (defined as surge capacity) and/or victims with unusual or highly specialized medical needs (defined as surge capability). In addition, public health and healthcare systems can expect incidents that significantly impact upon their usual operations. We have largely inculcated our populations to 'fall' onto hospitals and other healthcare delivery organizations in times of environmental duress.

HAZARD

These so-called 'mass effect' events can have devastating consequences for medically fragile segments of society and any of the multitudes of special needs populations.

The inability of special needs populations to access healthcare services can cause these populations to rapidly decompensate, producing a downstream surge of demand for acute care that can overwhelm local capabilities. This is a classic cascading affect that should be assumed under crisis conditions during a disaster. The first steps to address medical surge requirements and to build resiliency in the public health and healthcare infra-structure is to implement systems that can effectively manage medical and health response, as well as the development and maintenance of preparedness programmes focused on the public health and healthcare space.

The MSCC Management System describes a management methodology based on valid principles of emergency management and the Incident Command System (ICS). Public health and healthcare organizations can apply these principles to coordinate effectively with one another and to integrate with other response organizations that have established ICS and emergency management systems (fire service, law enforcement, etc.). At a minimum, this would help to reduce the notion of siloization previously mentioned and reduce the impact of C^2 fractionalization that occurs throughout the critical infrastructure sectors involved with disaster incident management.

 PEARL OF WISDOM

A 'commonalized' emergency management system for all response entities – public and private – is the ideal for managing any type of emergency.

The MSCC Management System also helps the public health and healthcare infrastructures to emplace a response architecture that is consistent with the National Incident Management System (NIMS), the over-arching national C^2 architecture that is delineated in the US National Response Framework.

The MSCC Management System describes a framework of coordination and integration across six tiers of response:

- **Management of Individual Healthcare Assets (Tier 1):**
  A well-defined ICS to collect and process information, to develop incident plans and to manage decisions is essential to maximize MSCC. Robust processes must be applicable both to traditional hospital participants and to other healthcare organizations that may provide 'hands-on' patient care in an emergency (e.g. outpatient clinics, community health centres, private physician offices and others). Thus, each healthcare asset must have information management processes to enable

integration among healthcare organizations (at Tier 2) and with higher management tiers.

- **Management of a Healthcare Coalition (Tier 2):** Coordination among local healthcare assets is critical to provide adequate and consistent care across an affected jurisdiction. The healthcare coalition provides a central integration mechanism for information sharing and management coordination among healthcare assets and also establishes an effective and balanced approach to integrating medical assets into the jurisdiction's ICS.
- **Jurisdiction Incident Management (Tier 3):** A jurisdiction's ICS integrates healthcare assets with other response disciplines to provide the structure and support needed to maximize MSCC. In certain events, the jurisdictional ICS promotes a unified incident command approach that allows multiple response entities, including public health and medicine, to assume significant management responsibility.
- **Management of State Response (Tier 4):** State Government participates in medical incident response across a range of capacities, depending on the specific event. The State may be the lead incident command authority, it may provide support to incidents managed at the jurisdictional (Tier 3) level, or it may coordinate multi-jurisdictional incident response. Important concepts are delineated to accomplish all of these missions, ensuring that the full range of State public health and medical resources is brought to bear to maximize MSCC.
- **Interstate Regional Management Coordination (Tier 5):** Effective mechanisms must be implemented to promote incident management coordination between affected States. This ensures consistency in regional response through coordinated incident planning, enhances information exchange between interstate jurisdictions and maximizes MSCC through interstate mutual aid and other support. Tier 5 incorporates existing instruments, such as the Emergency Management Assistance Compact (EMAC) (state-to-contiguous-state mutual aid and support agreements entered into for the purposes of providing

emergency response assets during large-scale disasters) and describes established incident command and mutual aid concepts to address these critical needs.

- **National Support to State and Jurisdiction Management (Tier 6):** Effective management processes at the State (Tier 4) and jurisdiction (Tier 3) levels facilitate the request, receipt and integration of national public health and healthcare resources to maximize MSCC. The national public health and healthcare response is described, emphasizing the management aspects that are important for state and local managers to understand (CNA Corporation, 2004).

To build on the baseline MSCC Management System model, it is suggested that three additional tiers be added (see Fig. 3.3).

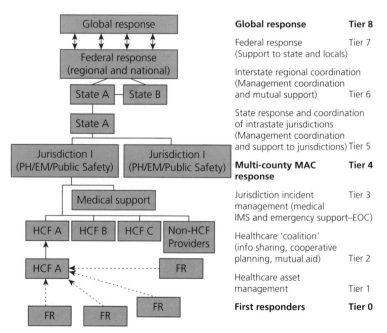

Fig. 3.3 MSCC management organization strategy revised. EM, emergency medicine; EOC, Emergency Operations Center; IMS, Incident Management System; FR, federal response; HCF, Healthcare Facility; MAC, Management Assistance Compacts; MSCC, Medical surge capacity and capability; PH, public health.

- **First Responders (Tier 0):** More often than not, first responders from local and regional Emergency Medical Services (EMS) are the first healthcare assets to make contact with affected populations. In as much, they are a 'first peer' through the aperture of a developing event. They can provide critical information to first receivers (Tier 1, Individual Healthcare Assets) and higher tiers to help prepare for mass casualty management. They are particularly important in event recognition involving the use of asymmetrical threat agents that may cause harm to the echelons above them without adequate warning from field assets (Okumura *et al.*, 2000).
- **Multi-county Medical Assistance Compacts (MAC) (new Tier 4):** Similar to state- emergency management assistance compacts (EMAC), these are pre-event deliberate planning initiatives that allow public health and healthcare resource sharing among geographically contiguous or proximal counties. This helps to preclude the collapse of any one or more individual healthcare assets by creating bleed-off resources to help absorb casualty loads.
- **Finally, Global Response (Tier 8):** Under certain scenarios (e.g. earthquakes, tsunamis, pandemic disease outbreaks), it is likely that public health and healthcare resources will be provided from other non-affected nations by way of humanitarian support and disaster assistance, or information shared that will aid in another country's ability to prepare for and prosecute incident management requirements.

In any effective plan, initiative or successful incident management mission, it is vital to observe the axiom of 'never plan or operate in a vacuum'. **All tiers must be fully coordinated if they hope to be successful**; as the scope and scale of the event becomes progressively larger, the importance of this requirement increases in proportional measure. Additionally, the MSCC Management System architecture needs to be completely transparent to and confluent with all non-medical incident response capabilities if the overall incident management mission is to be successful, since other critical infrastructure and key resource assets will be required to help support the public health and healthcare infrastructure. The processes that promote this coordination and integration enable public health and healthcare systems to move beyond their traditional support roles (for example, as an Emergency Support Function) and become competent participants in large-scale medical incident management.

● Practical applications

Building on the MSCC Management System as the under-pinning architecture for health and healthcare preparedness and response, the following theoretical application models are offered for consideration:

1. The Hospital Emergency Response Coalition (HERC) model hospital

The Hospital Emergency Response Coalition (HERC) Model was formed to address concerns about healthcare organization siloization and the lack of communicability among hospitals. Hospitals – especially those in the private, for-profit sector – are notoriously protective of their proprietary information. Since many of them are competing with one another for capturing market share among their catchment population, they are not in the general habit of facilitating the free and open sharing of information, hence, they generally lack any sort of 'network centricity' when it comes to collaborative planning for disaster response. This facilitates the placing of public health and healthcare resources into an 'at-risk' category during disasters, since the lack of collaboration and sharing of combined assets can facilitate their collapse as silos when severe environmental risk becomes evident.

In the case of the HERC initiative, local stakeholders recognized that this was a legitimate concern among the area healthcare organizations that supported them. Since they were in a particularly at-risk location (secondary to routine severe weather patterns) in the United States, they 'persuaded' the county hospital organizations to enter into a collaborative coalition for enhancing emergency response. The persuasion in this case was funding. Since facilitating this network-centric approach to planning was largely fear-driven, a portion of the catchment population to this particular set of regional assets decided to under-write the initiative and thus was born the HERC.

Although it's unusual and highly unrepresentative of how other coalitions might be formed for positive effect, the lessons of the model should not be lost. First off, the model borrows heavily from the 'Concentric Ring' concept of vaccination used to eradicate smallpox under the direction of Dr DA Henderson, but in reverse. Healthcare organizations within a geographically proximal position to one another enter into a network-centric, collaborative disaster preparedness network. As an 'event' unfolds from its locus to the nearest facilities, the networked hospitals essentially create internal pressure relief systems, allowing casualty streams to either flow out of or be directed directly to geographically distal facilities within the network, precluding any one facilities or group of facilities from collapse due to their inability to manage excess surge. This spread-loading of surge requirements creates an absorption model similar to concentric ring vaccination; that is – at least theoretically – by the time the most geographically distal locations have absorbed in the affected populations, the incident management mission for the affected population can be brought to a successful close.

The challenges of the HERC model are not dissimilar to effectively emplacing the tenets of the MSCC Management System. Getting public health and healthcare organizations alone to communicate effectively with one another is of itself no small task. Dr Lenny Marcus at the Harvard School of Public Health has suggested that the medical and public health communities' *writ large* suffers from what he refers to as the 'Dilemma of the Cube'. The cube in this case is in fact a shared mission, that of the health, safety and survivability of their communities. Both communities 'peer' or 'reach' into the cube to 'grasp' their mission, but the disparate differences in the perspectives of the two communities causes them to 'see' something different within the mission space and the silos are maintained. Dr Marcus and his colleagues at Harvard maintain that it is only the 'meta-leaders' within one or both of the communities who grasp the true commonality of the mission and the need for ongoing collaboration. The same concept is *apropos* to healthcare and hospital-based organizations. Until they peer through the common aperture of the mission and agree that they are all striving for the same net result, we will not see substantive increases in surge capacity preparedness and the ability to deal adequately with large-scale events.

2. The 'Location of Opportunity Surge Capacity' Model

The next theoretical application model is referred to as the 'Location of Opportunity Surge Capacity Model' (see Fig. 3.4). Here, we assume that the hospital or medical treatment facility locations of a particular geographic location (e.g. town, city, county) are, in fact, static relative to a capitated level of organic surge capacity. In this case, we recognize in advance of a disaster that there are scenarios (i.e. towards the high-operational to strategic in terms of impact) that will inherently tax their ability to provide surge to the point of near-term collapse.

In this model, there are two important assumptions to consider:

- The most valuable assets to the healthcare organizations are not their static space facilities or limited resources pools. **The most important assets to the healthcare organizations are the professional competencies of their provider base** and these assets have to be protected so that they can become 'directive' resources to managing large surge populations that will require their expertise during a disaster.

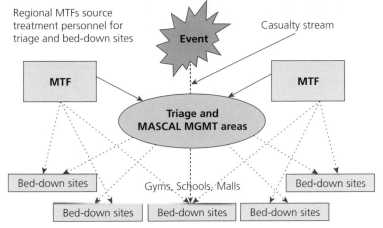

Fig. 3.4 Additional CONOPS 'ideas'. CONOPS, concept of operations; MASCAL MGMT, mass casualty management; MTF, medical treatment facility (hospitals). Bed-down sites are minimal care beds; heavy reliance on self- and buddy aid.

- It follows that **there will be a diminishment of the standard of care** that is inversely proportional to the magnitude of the event and that during the event, non-traditional provider populations (e.g. para-professionals, family, neighbours and surviving well populations) will have to be leveraged under the direction of credentialed providers to support the affected population.

In the pre-event phase of this model; public health and health-care planners, working in close collaboration with regional disaster management officials, coordinate the sighting of locations of opportunity for managing surge requirements. Fixed facilities such as schools, malls and gymnasia are designated as the surge locations. It is even possible (and highly recommended) that these facilities be assigned an acuity value based on triage categories (e.g. acute, immediate, delayed, expectant).

As an event begins to unfold, designated disaster response personnel from the public health and healthcare communities set up an immediate triage filter in a safety zone outside of the locus of the event and begin to process patients to the surge

PEARL OF WISDOM

Baseline medical resources to support surge locations can and should be stockpiled, so that there are communal assets that can be drawn on to use during a disaster. Most communities around the world rely on just-in-time inventories; the failure to stockpile even the barest of medical necessities such as bandages, iv and resuscitative fluids, disinfectant products and cots can prove disastrous.

locations of opportunity. Doing this outside of the existent static hospitals facilities reduces the risk of providers being overwhelmed and protects them as the community's most important asset during a disaster.

3. The Regional Public Health and Healthcare Surge Capacity Model

The third theoretical application presented is the 'Regional Public Health and Medical Surge Capacity Model'. This construct assumes a large-scale event well outside the ability of tactical or low-operational management scale. This further assumes that there will be multi-jurisdictional management requirements that are needed to prosecute the public health and healthcare incident management missions. This is the model truest to the 'event of national significance' or national mass casualty incident paradigm. The diagram in Figure 3.5 presents an omni-directional pattern for incident management. Note that it is easily capable of being scaled to a multi-directional pattern as event expansion occurs.

In this case, the locus of the event is assumed to be a 'hot zone' which may present further danger to directly affected populations if they are not removed from the area of impact. Likewise, it should be assumed that sending anyone into the hot zone could prove to be dangerous for a wide variety of reasons (e.g. disease exposure, hazardous material exposure, risk of exposure to dangerous natural elements, lawlessness). In any case, it would be unwise to send credentialed providers in to this area to perform search and rescue and initial patient encounters. Leveraging trained rescue personnel and/or low-level medical personnel (e.g. EMTs, EMS responders) to conduct this mission would be recommended.

Collected victims would be removed from the hot zone to casualty collection zone within a location marked as the 'FEBA,' a term derived from the military and standing for 'forward edge of the battle area'. This is the location where victims would be married to the first layer of transportation assets (e.g. ground ambulances, rotary wing lift if available, other overland movement assets) and sent to 'temporary medical operations support areas' or 'TMOSAs', which serve as the disaster triage filters to sort patients based on acuity categories. TMOSAs should be set up sufficiently distal to an event to preclude degradation but at the same time be proximal enough to ensure adequate time is available to enhance survivability.

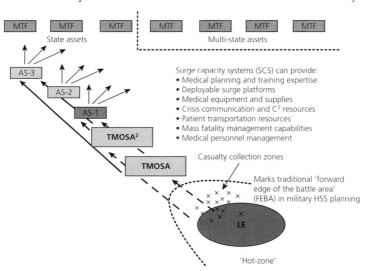

Fig. 3.5 Catastrophic Casuality Event (CCE) Medical Planning Support Construct. AS, acuity station; HSS, health services support; LE, localus of event; MTF, medical treatment facility (fixed); TMOSA, temporary medical operations support area (triage filter).

Once patients are given a triage category, they are married to the second layer of transportation assets and retrograded to designated acuity stations, which as Figure 3.5 shows are proportionally distal to the TMOSAs (i.e. 'immediate' category is closest). Once stabilized at the acuity stations, patients are married to the third layer of transportation and finally retrograded to fixed medical treatment facilities that have been identified as capable of absorbing the surge requirements, either at the state or multi-state level.

● Managing the masses in a behavioural model of surge

The final theoretical approach addresses the incredible but clearly literature-supported 100 to 1 ratio represented by the behavioural model of surge. This augmented surge is untenable with traditional resource-based surge planning. An understanding that Surge Capacity and Surge Capability represent separate and distinct aspects of the surge management equation, however, lends to a behavioural model for managing mass casualty surge and by extension mass fatality surge.

Similar to Shultz's deconstruction of the historical components of surge, Shultz examined needs-based options for the disposition of surge. Shultz *et al.* (2006) described, and several metropolitan programmes including the HERC and the Minneapolis Metropolitan Hospital Compact adopted, the Hospital Based Support Center and the Free Standing Family Center as diversion sites for the psychologically injured, 'co-arrivals' and 'searching citizens.'

Shultz and Ramirez (2007) determined that direction of the psychologically injured patients to a Hospital Based Support Center immediately following the determination of medical stability by an emergency medical screening examination reduces patient surge in the medical care areas by 80 per cent. Ramirez subsequently found that when the Free Standing Family Center is outside the secure common mechanical facilities of the main hospital building or completely off hospital property, EMTALA concerns no longer apply. Overall the combined use of the Free Standing Family Center and the Hospital Based Support Center reduced patient care surge demand (physical and psychological injury care) by 75 per cent while reducing medical care surge demand (physical injury care) by 95 per cent.

THINKING POINT

'There are risks and costs to a program of action, but they are far less than the long-range risks and costs of comfortable inaction.' President John F. Kennedy

Summary

In his 2004 book *American Soldier*, retired US General Tommy Franks referred to the events of 9/11 as a 'crease in history'. The world was one way before that day and it will never be the same again. In the mid-nineteenth century, there was a popular pseudoscientific/philosophical movement called 'Catastrophism,' which essentially theorized that there are events of such magnitude as to alter the course of the universe, the earth, or human and animal species. There are certainly events throughout the course of history that give merit to the context of this philosophy.

In modern times, the fact is that acts of terrorism, horrific natural disasters and monumentally egregious man-made errors and mistakes will create situations that fundamentally tax to the point of disruption or collapse our ability to maintain the homeostasis of our communities, nations and regions. These events *can* and *will* influence the course of history and the scale and scope of their impact may be adjudicated on our ability to effectively emplace the response and recovery controls emerging in the discipline of emergency and disaster management.

This chapter seeks to provide its readers with some theoretical and practical skill-sets to help improve the 'posture of preparedness' for the nations and regions they serve. It seeks to engage them in the understanding that the potential for calamity is omnipresent and that only by turning full-face to the challenges of these threats can we hope to improve our chances of survival and recovery. Of paramount importance, it seeks to create the linkage among the Nations that the burden of catastrophe is one to be shared and that networked response architecture enhances the fabric of safety in the common society of the human species.

REFERENCES

The CNA Corporation *Medical Surge Capacity and Capability: a management system for integrating medical and health resources during large-scale emergencies,* CNA, Washington, DC, 2004.

Davis TE. *Autopsy of a Mega-Casualty Event: what are the principles?* Seminar Series, Centers for Disease Control, Atlanta, 2004.

Okumura T, Suzuki K, Ichimatsu S, Takasu N, Fuiji C, Kohama A. Lessons learned from Tokyo Sarin attack. *Pre-hospital Disaster Medicine* 2000; **18** (3): 189–91.

Schultz JM and Ramirez MA. Surge Sort Support: disaster *behavioral health for healthcare providers* [Seminar Series]. University of Miami, Disaster and Extreme Event Preparedness Center, 2007.

Shultz JM, Espinel Z, Cohen RE *et al. Disaster Behavioural Health: all-hazards training.* University of Miami, DEEP Center, Miami, 2003.

Shultz JM, Espinel Z, Cohen RE *et al. Surge, Sort and Support: disaster behavioural health for healthcare providers.* University of Miami, DEEP Center, Miami, 2006.

4 Classification of disasters

RMF Gill

● What is a disaster?

A definition is a good place to start any classification, especially for a word in such common use. Many of us use the word in everyday parlance and the media are prone to use 'disaster' or 'disastrous' to describe any minor setback. Even at a more serious level, the term 'disaster planning' is often loosely used to describe the emergency planning in hospitals, with which most of us are familiar, now widespread since it was directed by the Civil Contingencies Act 2004.

Looking back at Chapter 3, we can see a clear view of what a disaster is *not*. **It is not a major incident**. These are defined in NHS Emergency Planning Guidance 2005 as: 'Any occurrence that presents serious threat to the health of the community, disruption to the service or causes (or is likely to cause) such numbers or types of casualties as to require special arrangements to be implemented by hospitals, ambulance trusts or primary care organisations'. Equally **it is not an accident**: 'An event which results in casualties where the social fabric remains intact and the community is able to cope'.

A definition we can more readily identify within the context of this book is a: 'great, sudden misfortune resulting in loss of life, serious injury and property destruction' (Orlowski, 1988), but this raises the question of how many deaths and injuries.

This sort of detail is much sought after in a developing disaster and helps to secure both headlines and money for action. While in the past people have categorized disasters according to the numbers of casualties, deaths, or refugees, the question for us as medical personnel is probably more 'Am I needed?'

L LEARNING POINT

A disaster, while not a major incident or an accident, may be defined as: 'A disruption of the human ecology, which the affected community cannot overcome with its own resources' (Reis and Dolev, 1989). It is the need for external assistance which is relevant.

You may wonder if the definition really matters. **The key is the consequence** – the need for external assistance, which is how we come to be involved. There are plenty of definitions of disasters to be found, and precisely which one you use is not critical, but it is important to be confident about the words you use, as the international agencies, the humanitarian workers you deal with and donors who fund disaster relief will want to be precise about the situation.

● The scale of disasters

When considering scale we typically think first of the number of dead in the transport disasters or terrorist attacks we have seen in the developed world, such as the 31 deaths in the Paddington Rail Crash (1999), or the 3232 deaths of the 2001 World Trade Center attacks. Major natural disasters are not common in the developed world, but recent examples include 1836 deaths in Hurricane Katrina in 2005 and the 6348 deaths of the 1995 Kobe earthquake.

The scale of natural disasters in the developing world is so completely different as to be hard to comprehend. They do not compare with infectious disease as causes of global mortality, but their impact can be gleaned from some broad comparisons of scale. Individual examples of major disasters include the 1970 Bhola cyclone in Bangladesh (then E. Pakistan) – 300 000 deaths; the 1976 Tangshan earthquake – 255 000 deaths; the 1985 Nevada del Ruiz eruption in Columbia – 25 000 deaths and the 2004 Indian Ocean Tsunami – 225 000 deaths.

Looking at the overall picture, in each of the decades of the 1970s and 1980s, roughly one million people died in natural disasters worldwide and two billion people (almost a third of the world's population) were significantly affected. The vast majority of these were in the developing world. In the 1990s the numbers of dead reduced by about a half, but the total numbers affected have risen to 2½ billion, and the economic costs have risen from an estimated $40 billion per year in the 1980s to $145 billion in 2004.

Despite the publicity that disasters in the developed world such as Hurricane Katrina attract, **90 per cent of natural disasters occur in the developing world** and the impact there is much greater, both in human cost and impact on the economy. The economic cost of disasters in the developing world is typically lower, as there is less expensive property and infrastructure to be damaged, but the cost as a proportion of the national wealth is much greater. For example, the cost of Hurricane Katrina in 2005 was about 1 per cent of the gross domestic product (GDP – the total market value of all final

HAZARD

Consequences of disasters
Death
Disability
Disease
Food and resource scarcity
Population movement

goods and services produced within a country in a year) of the USA, but in Honduras Hurricane Mitch in 1998 cost 41 per cent of GDP, and the cost of the 2004 Tsunami in the worst-hit Indonesian province of Acheh was equivalent to 97 per cent of its GDP.

● Consequences

There are various ways of thinking about different sorts of disaster. The number of deaths is often the most-quoted consequence and is certainly a measure of impact. As medical staff, although the mortality rate is a vital indicator of outcome and of healthcare needs, the number of overall deaths is usually a secondary consideration, as we are concentrating on the survivors. After all, we have little to offer the dead and diagnostic pathological examination is likely to be redundant. Forensic pathology investigation may, however, be a major issue in conflict, where war crimes are often suspected or alleged, but it is a specialist skill and highly politically sensitive, and emergency medical providers will generally try to distance themselves from such work. There is often concern about the risk of disease being spread by dead bodies which have not been disposed of properly. This is a very real risk in a cholera outbreak, when they can be a major source of contamination – this is one of the few occasions when you may need to over-ride normal cultural practices, as bodies of cholera victims are best decontaminated and buried as quickly as possible, rather than returning to families for traditional ceremonies. It is also a risk in outbreaks of plague and typhus but, otherwise, the public health risks of corpses do not usually take precedence over the needs of the

PEARL OF WISDOM

Concentrate on the survivors, and be less focused on the dead.

living, including their need to grieve and handle the dead in a culturally appropriate manner (Morgan, 2006). All these are reasons to be less focused on the dead.

On the other hand, there are areas of concern to us. A community will be dependent on the survivors for recovery and the pattern and extent of death thus has an impact on the ability of the community to recover. Broadly speaking, in many natural disasters such as famine, the weakest are at greatest risk of death, potentially leaving a comparatively healthy survivor population to recover. In conflict, on the other hand, the young and active are more likely to be killed, detained, maimed or injured, leaving a more dependent population, with a diminished ability to help itself.

Death also leaves survivors grieving, but it is hard for us to help this. Grief and reactions to bereavement are highly culturally specific. Attitudes and expressions of grief vary greatly, and can cause misunderstanding, and external intervention carries the risk of making things worse. The complex nature of transcultural psychiatry makes mental health-related issues especially hard to manage (Médecins Sans Frontières, 1997) and psychological aspects are covered in Chapter 9. Unless you are fortunate enough to be working with healthcare workers with highly detailed local knowledge, this is something you will have to watch out for, but may find difficult to get involved with.

Finally, the highlight on the numbers of dead, albeit potentially distracting from the needs of the living, brings one benefit. Although a great deal of energy can be expended on arguing over numbers of deaths, typically for political or ideological reasons (Holocaust denial is perhaps the most obvious, but there are also debates on many other topics, such as over the numbers of deaths predicted following radiation exposure from Chernobyl), the level of interest means that the figure for deaths is likely to be known with a much greater degree of accuracy than others, such as overall numbers of injured, victims of disease, or refugees. While comparing different disaster circumstances is fraught with pitfalls, it nevertheless provides the single most accurate benchmark.

The long-term impact of disability on a survivor population is also important. The fate of mine victims has been publicized in recent years, but there are multiple causes of disability in disasters. Apart from the consequences for the disabled individual, who may be unable to earn a living or subsist and may be marginalized, the disabled may be unable to assist in the recovery of the community.

The impact of disease can be immense, and dealing with disease is central to much of disaster management. In this context it is its contribution both to disability and susceptibility to further consequences that is relevant, particularly malnutrition and other disease.

All of these consequences but particularly death or the threat of death (most acutely in concerns for personal security), food and resource scarcity and population movement, have the potential to feed on each other to cause a cycle or spiral of catastrophic decline. We will look at this below.

 LEARNING POINTS

Types of disaster

Natural

- Famine
- Drought
- Geophysical
- Earthquake
- Volcano
- Wind and water
  - Flood
  - Hurricane/cyclone/typhoon
  - Tsunami
- Wildfire

Man-made
- Transport
  - Air
  - Sea
  - Land
- Industrial
  - Chemical
  - Nuclear
  - Biological
- Conflict

Combination emergencies
- Simple
- Complex

● Categorization of disasters

Disasters are readily classified into natural, man-made and combinations of the two.

Natural disasters

Natural disasters can be defined as geological, atmospheric, hydrological and biological, but one event frequently leads to another (for example a tropical cyclone – atmospheric event – leading to storm surge and/or flooding – hydrological event). In any case it is the consequences rather than the physical characteristics which are of greater concern to us and so we have classified them (see Learning Points above) in a way that associates cause and effect.

Natural disasters have received greater public attention in the last few years, partly because they are seen as more amenable to intervention and prevention, especially since the 2004 tsunami raised awareness and triggered global interest in early warning systems for tsunamis and other events. The other main factor has been increased concern that global climate change will increase the frequency and impact of climatic disasters. Later we take the example of tropical cyclones.

Man-made disasters

Transport accidents causing mass casualties in developed countries are familiar as they are regularly described in the media. Industrial disasters are also familiar. Among the better-known examples of the differing types of industrial disasters are the chemical disaster at the Union Carbide plant in Bhopal in 1984, killing up to 5000, and the nuclear disaster at Chernobyl in 1986, causing about 60 short-term deaths and possibly several thousand premature deaths over subsequent decades. Among the reasons these and others (such as the Three Mile Island nuclear accident, which caused no immediate deaths) are well-known, is that they have been dramatized on screen and/or in print, including the 2007 Booker-shortlisted *Animal's People*, by Indra Sinha, about Bhopal. The biological leak of anthrax at Sverdlovsk in 1979, killing about 60, is less well-known and may be the only example of a man-made industrial biological disaster.

With the exception of Bhopal, we can see that the numbers of immediate deaths in transport and industrial disasters and accidents are small in comparison with natural disasters in the developing world. Comprehensive regulations and controls are in place in most countries to limit the impact and risk of industrial disasters and accidents, which are closely linked to environmental concerns. The financial and legal implications of failure mean that the vast majority of companies and operators have strong incentives to comply. This field is an extensive area of its own, which is well-covered elsewhere, so here we will concentrate on natural disasters and complex emergencies.

Example – tropical cyclones

As an example of natural disaster and of disasters in general, we can look at tropical cyclones in the Bay of Bengal. Tropical cyclones are low pressure storm systems with strong winds and heavy rain, which form in susceptible areas in the tropics. The most severe tropical cyclones are known as typhoons in the Northwest Pacific and hurricanes in the Northeast Pacific and Atlantic.

The principal effects of a tropical cyclone are:

- Storm surges, generated by strong winds – the sea level rises near the coast, inundating low lying areas, drowning people and live-stock, destroying crops and damaging soil. This is the most destructive element.
- Very strong winds damage buildings, communication systems and trees, causing death and destruction.
- Heavy and prolonged rains, causing river floods and more inundation.
- Drinking water sources are polluted by inundation causing disease.

The characteristics of cyclones enable them to be tracked using current meteorological technology, and observation and experience allows their behaviour and path to be predicted (with a degree of error – about 200 km in a 24-hour forecast). The prediction, combined with the communication systems available, dictates the amount of time people have to react and thus influences the actions that can be taken to manage the hazard. These include construction to resist or escape floods, flood defences, warning systems to rapidly spread messages and training, so that people know what to expect and what to do.

We can see how a structured approach can be taken to dealing with disaster hazard, using tropical cyclones as an example (see Hazard box below).

Putting all this together, we can see how the design of a **disaster management plan**, still using tropical cyclone as an example (see Learning Points below), depends on understanding the characteristics and effects of the disaster, the capabilities of technology and the ability of the society to react.

HAZARD

Phases of tropical cyclone danger

- Threat – living in an area where tropical cyclones can occur.
- Warning – from meteorological and communication systems.
- Impact – the acute phase when a disaster occurs.
- Assessment/Inventory – assessing the damage.
- Rescue – assistance from those on the spot.
- Relief – assistance from outside.
- Rehabilitation – trying to restore normality.

CASE STUDY

Bangladesh cyclone

In Bangladesh, cyclone warning systems include radio transmission to the district offices of The Red Crescent, from which a network of tens of up to thousands of volunteers is activated. These volunteers set out on bicycles, equipped with megaphones, to deliver the warning by the simplest and most direct means, so that people can move to shelters. Other critical elements of preparation include extensive training, both of the volunteer network and of all people in the vulnerable areas so they know what the warnings mean and what action to take; the building and stocking of the shelters; and arrangements to transport people to safe areas in a timely manner.

This system was used when Bangladesh was affected by Cyclone Sidr in November 2007. As a result the death toll was contained at about 3000, instead of potentially hundreds of thousands. Millions were homeless but many people were saved and able to start recovery and rebuilding.

● Conflict

Although conflict is covered in greater detail in other chapters a few factors need to be considered here. In particular, it is the social and political nature of war, as described most famously by Clausewitz, which is relevant. The nature of war as a social and political activity means that it is intimately bound up with all aspects of the life of the society, and thus any activity carried on in that society relates to the war in some way. It follows that providers of medical aid (or other humanitarian support) will not be seen as independent of conflict, but as factors in it, or as participants. This is deeply disturbing to most humanitarian workers and especially to medical personnel, who naturally try to manage the patient independently of conflict or other non-clinical factors. Many of the provisions of the Law of Armed Conflict are intended to support humanitarian and medical activity and in conventional wars between countries this is often fairly effective, but in civil war there is much less protection.

For us, the key point beyond the unpredictability of war (and the 'friction' described by Clausewitz which makes everything more difficult) is the way in which people are involved at every level, as perpetrators, victims, objects and targets. Especially in a civil war, a victim of war who is treated successfully may return immediately to action to fight. A fighter who is fixed on the rightness of his cause may well see his opponents as legitimate targets whatever their condition, perhaps because he believes them to be terrorists or responsible for atrocities.

HAZARD

It is a comparatively short step for a fighter in a civil war to see those who aid his opponents (including by giving them medical aid or treatment), as legitimate targets. This is unpalatable, not to say frightening, but it is a risk of which we must be aware, even if we do not let it prevent us from getting involved. This is not only for our own personal security (pretty relevant of itself – killed or injured staff cannot help others), but also because it puts our patients at increased risk.

The sort of case outlined above is extreme, although there are examples from the former Yugoslavia and Chechnya, but the fact remains that even in less brutal conflicts the provision of medical or other humanitarian aid cannot confidently be assumed to be perceived as a neutral act, irrespective of the spirit in which it is given.

● Complex emergencies

The most demanding disasters of all are 'complex emergencies', described by the UN Inter-Agency Standing Committee (IASC) in 1994 as:

'…a humanitarian crisis in a country, region or society where there is total or considerable breakdown of authority resulting from internal or external conflict and which requires an international response that goes beyond the mandate or capacity of any single agency and/or the ongoing United Nations country program.'

It is these large-scale, frequently intractable crises, that spring to mind when we think about humanitarian disasters. Classic examples from the 1990s, some continuing directly or through secondary crises to this day, include Somalia, Kosovo, and the genocide, civil war, and refugee crisis in Rwanda (and subsequent enduring conflict in the Democratic Republic of the Congo).

It was stated above that the differing consequences of disasters can fuel each other in a cyclical catastrophic manner. To look at an example, when there is conflict in a state, refugees are highly likely to try to escape it by crossing the border. If they are in large numbers, they will impose a drain on resources in the host country and if they become established, they may become a focus for further conflict. This might be external, possibly by setting up exile groups which attack the country of origin or they may act as a magnet for aggression from the country of origin. Or it might be internal, triggering new power struggles within the host country. The history of the Rwandan and associated conflicts in the Great Lakes region of central Africa offers numerous examples.

Beyond the obvious tragedy of spreading conflict, the particular implications for us are in the attitude to humanitarian agencies. Any of the above outcomes are likely to be unpopular with the host country, who may adopt policies to encourage refugees to return home. In enlightened countries these may be moderate and fully integrated with the approach of humanitarian agencies. In less tolerant countries there may be greater pressure for refugees to return hastily, including by violence or the threat of violence and they may look unfavourably on humanitarian agencies providing aid to refugees, to the extent that they interfere or seek to prevent them operating. At the very least there will probably be banditry and freelance criminality, which flourish in the lawless conditions of civil conflict. These may target humanitarian agencies and their equipment. A failed state may be powerless to protect agencies rather than able to deliberately target them but the effect is much the same. All these are classic characteristics of complex emergencies.

Above all, in complex emergencies it is the effect of conflict and violence which is central to both the impact of the crises and their insoluble nature, but the combination and interplay of factors involved makes them resistant to conventional peacemaking and peacekeeping approaches (which are themselves difficult enough to accomplish). Successful resolution will invariably depend on an approach which includes all actors – political (states and internal power factions), intergovernmental bodies, non-governmental organizations and aid agencies – and typically involves difficult political decisions, such as leaving some parties unsatisfied. All too often this is not achievable, or at least not in the short term, and a cycle of conflict and catastrophe is established which lasts for years and years.

It is against this sort of appalling prospect that efforts to resolve any complex emergency should be considered. While the 'big picture' of the international political perspective might seem to be immaterial to those of us healthcare workers involved in the immediate care of the suffering, it is crucial to have realistic expectations and some sense of what is achievable. Inevitably and sadly, this involves accepting less than the ideal.

● Disasters and development

A simplistic view is sometimes taken that there is a clear distinction between a disaster, when something suddenly goes wrong, and development work, where a measured and planned approach is taken to promoting economic development and welfare. Although elements of this persist, for example in the approach to funding, this has been widely challenged (Sollis, 1994).

The cyclone preparedness work in Bangladesh is an obvious example of effective development, but other links can be found through UN activity, particularly the International

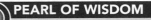

PEARL OF WISDOM

Development projects frequently have the prevention or mitigation of disasters in mind. The poorest people with little or no reserves of money or stocks will be the most vulnerable to even a small threat to their livelihoods; a disaster has the potential to halt or wreck a development project, but **effective development can improve resilience to disasters.**

Strategy for Disaster Reduction. This was already focusing on planning for disasters and addressing vulnerability, especially through technical measures, before the 2004 tsunami. Since then there has been a great increase in awareness in the developed world. As the Bangladesh example shows, technical measures alone are not enough and there is considerable debate between differing interests which are competing for funding.

The reality is that disasters and development activity are certainly inter-related, but the relationship is no simpler than any other in the intricate interaction between factors in complex emergencies. While we often think of a disaster disrupting development activity, it could also work the other way: looking at a project such as a dam on a major river flowing across a continent (for example on the scale of the Three Gorges Dam on the Yangtse river), we can start to see how a major development project might have a differential economic impact, which could destabilize relations between different nations, tribes or socio-economic groups and create tensions which could lead to unrest in an unstable society.

There is another aspect, which is to do with releasing money to assist. Past major disasters have stimulated specific funding campaigns, looking for public donations. This still occurs but the vast majority of funding now comes from governments, or inter-government organizations such as the European Union. This also applies to money for development projects, which are usually plentiful in the countries that suffer from disasters.

The significance of the distinction is that disaster money typically comes with fewer strings attached – the donors understand that there is no time for submitting detailed plans for approval, or placing constraints such as specifying how projects are to be delivered, as is normal in development projects. Disaster funding thus has benefits for agencies receiving it, as they get more freedom of action in how they spend it, even if they may still have to account for it afterwards.

Disaster relief can either hinder or help long-term development. One of the most obvious risks is of diverting funding to short-term disaster relief. Another is of generating a dependency which cannot be sustained.

CLINICAL CONSIDERATIONS

In a refugee camp during conflict it may be necessary to set up a medical facility providing surgery if existing facilities are unable to cope. If the flow of conflict casualties reduces, or there is spare capacity, the facility may attract patients with general surgical problems, or cases such as obstetric emergencies. If there are no other surgical facilities in the area **a dependency may be created**. Similarly, if patients are attracted away from existing facilities (perhaps by providing free treatment as opposed to fee-charging), **the local health economy may be destabilized**. This risk is present in all disaster relief activities, for example in food relief and is thus best managed as part of the wider overall disaster relief plan. The lead agencies will play a key role in coordinating and advising on this risk.

● Conclusion

Disasters, and especially complex emergencies, are multifaceted and difficult to understand, particularly when you are intimately involved in them. A systematic approach to organizing thoughts is vital to enable us to take a logical approach to the vast array of factors and detailed problems which present. Being able to classify different forms of disaster and relate them to their outcomes is the first step.

Summary

- Disasters have a massive impact world-wide.
- The burden falls most heavily on those least able to deal with it.
- Disasters are readily classified into natural, man-made and combinations of the two.
- Complex emergencies are especially intractable.
- Understanding the nature of differing types of disaster helps us to develop our approach to managing them.
- In particular, appreciating some of the convoluted factors involved in complex emergencies, as a result of conflict, is essential to effective operating and survival.

REFERENCES

Médecins Sans Frontières. *Refugee Health – an approach to emergency situations*. Macmillan, London, 1997.

Morgan O. (ed.) *Management of Dead Bodies After Disasters: a field manual for first responders*. PAHO, Washington DC, 2006.

Orlowski J. Chapter in Baskett P and Weller R. (eds) *Medicine for Disasters*. Wright, Oxford, 1988.

Reis ND and Dolev E. (eds) *Manual of Disaster Medicine: Civilian and Military*. Springer-Verlag, New York, 1989.

Sollis P. The relief-development continuum: some notes on rethinking for civilian victims of conflict. *Journal of International Affairs* 1994; **47**: 451–71.

5

Pre- and post-deployment

Ken Roberts

● Destination and decisions

So you want to be involved in this sort of deployment? Think about your motivation: are you intending to do this through altruism, a sense of guilt, arrogance or adventure (or a combination of them)? Do not take the decision to do so lightly; as discussed elsewhere in this chapter you are highly likely to be part of a team, so you owe it to them (and your potential clients) to become involved for the right reasons.

Find out as much as you can about the organization you will be working for, especially its ethos, aims and reputation. The most reputable ones have open and honest websites, which you should use as the basis for more directed queries to the organization itself. Clearly, this is a two-way street, and (as you might expect) you will be subject to a selection process to ensure that you are suited for your intended deployment.

You will obviously need to establish that you possess the appropriate qualities and skills to meet your part in the expected mission. Again, these will be set and validated by your potential employing organization, although you can get a good idea of what these requirements are likely to be by referring to the organization's website and by researching what the expected type of deployment will be by looking at websites such as ReliefWeb (www.reliefweb.org). See the end of this chapter for more examples.

Also, using some of the sources of information discussed later in this chapter, find out as much as you can about the climate, topography and cultural issues involved with your destination, and judge if you are suited for the deployment. Finally, meet the other potential members of your team, and decide if you could work and live with them for a significant period of time under stressful conditions.

● Team selection, building and maintenance

The provision of effective medical care to disasters is essentially a team effort, since no single individual can provide all of the skills involved. As will be discussed, although true teams can be a very efficient type of group, they can be relatively delicate, especially during the early stages of their formation and require nurturing and maintenance. This is important, given that teams for this type of work are frequently formed at relatively short notice.

Teams and groups

A *team* (Adair, 1984) is essentially a *group* of willing and trained individuals who are:

- united around a common goal
- dependent upon each other to achieve that goal
- structured to work together
- empowered to implement decisions
- have shared responsibility for their task

The team itself is important, since (in addition to providing an appropriate mix of skills it):

- meets the psychosocial needs of its members and, once formed, can be relatively self-sustaining and satisfying;
- provides mutual support to its members;

- enables division of tasks amongst its members;
- can produce originality.

Groups are characterized by an evolutionary life-cycle (Handy, 1988), which must be understood if they are to deliver their task effectively without damaging their members. The stages of group evolution are summarized in Table 5.1.

Table 5.1 Life-cycle of groups

Stage	Characteristics	Outputs
Forming	Shyness, uncertainty, tentative	Little visible output Members are attempting to orientate themselves within the group
Storming	More open, complaining, criticizing, disagreeing, questioning of goals	Little visible output Members are confronting others within the group
Norming	Resolution of internal conflicts, division of responsibilities within group being resolved, emergence of group norms	Little visible output Nature of the group beginning to emerge
Performing	Collaboration, commitment, self-regulation	Group productivity increases. Group has evolved into a *team*
Dissolving	Sense of loss and lack of worth	When tight-knit groups/teams dissolve Little visible output

The potential risk in the evolution of the team (and the time taken for the team to form) can be reduced by a number of considerations.

Team selection

Procedures must be put into place to ensure that the appropriate individuals are selected for the team. Although, clearly, this will be on the basis of the skills required, this should not be the only criterion. It is important that team players with an enthusiasm for the task are chosen, and any selection procedure must take this and any health considerations into account.

Team building

Teams must have mutually agreed ground rules if they are to thrive and be effective. These should include:

- the recognition of equal respect for all members;
- the recognition and acceptance of differences between individuals (whether that be on the basis of gender, religion or ethnicity);
- the absolute intolerance of non-team behaviour, such as dishonesty and inappropriate sexual behaviour.

Furthermore, everyone needs to understand and accept procedures within the team for emergencies and for the reporting of perceived grievances and difficulties.

Team training

The team needs to be confident in its individual and collective competence and this can be nurtured by appropriate training. This should not merely involve ensuring that individuals' professional skills are kept up to date, but should also include basic survival techniques such as safety, personal and collective hygiene drills and defensive driving. **Training in the correct use of protective equipment and communications systems is vital** and a degree of cross-training between team members can be useful.

Team maintenance

It is important that all members of the team are aware of its mission, goals and what outputs it should be achieving. Everyone needs to be aware of their contribution to the overall effort and what their responsibilities are. The team can be further maintained by a fair division of tasks (i.e. everyone does some of the seemingly menial chores, irrespective of who they are). Regular progress discussions (What have we done today? What went right? What went wrong? What will we do tomorrow?) are useful, provided they are conducted in a non-confrontational way. A good idea is to structure these around communal meal times, when everyone can relax somewhat.

The morale and cohesion of the team will also be enhanced by attention to administrative issues such as the provision of contact with home (by mail or telecommunications). Leadership (not necessarily in the traditional hierarchical sense) is an important 'glue' for any team, although these aspects would be the subject of a separate book!

Dissolving teams

It is important to reduce the stress of the grieving process by dissolving teams sensitively. Members should be encouraged to celebrate the team's achievements and to keep in touch after the team has dissolved. Further issues of this nature will be discussed later in this chapter.

THINKING POINTS

- Think about a successful team that you have been involved with in the past. What characteristics set it apart for you?
- Consider your own character (objectively, please!). What personal traits do you possess that would be beneficial in maintaining a team ethos? What traits could be seen to be negative to a team and how would you modify your behaviour accordingly?

● Planning tools

As already described, it is almost inevitable that you will be working as part of a team during this type of deployment. Remember that an important characteristic of the team is that it is based around a common goal. An essential component of this is to plan what the team intends to do and agree on how to achieve it (Hodgkinson and Stewart, 1991). Without this essential preparation for coordinated activity, it is more likely that the team will fail in its task, which is unacceptable. **Even in an emergency situation, there will always be time to plan** and this time will never be wasted (Lloyd Roberts, 2005).

PEARL OF WISDOM

- Prior
- Preparation and
- Planning
- Prevent
- Pathetically
- Poor
- Performance

Principles of effective planning

- **The aim** – You must accurately identify and define exactly what you intend to do. Identify only one aim, to keep things simple and to avoid the possibility of confusion.
- **Time and distance** – Try to estimate how long it will take to complete your aim, taking into account such factors as travel time (and what would affect it such as travelling conditions and the distances involved). Mentally rehearse the task and try to imagine all of the practical issues involved, including what could go wrong and how that would affect your ability to meet the aim. You may find that you are unlikely to meet your aim in the time available to you, in which case you may need to revise it to make it more achievable.
- **Administration and logistics** – Think of all the things that you need to put in place to make your plan work. This will include estimating how many people you will need and of what skills mix and bear in mind what other tasks they may have carried out recently, to avoid them becoming overly fatigued. Identify what task-specific equipment you will require (and don't forget to check that it is working) and also what general support items (food, water, shelter and communications, for example) will need to be taken. Clearly, if other vehicle transport is required, it will be necessary to confirm its availability, serviceability and whether you will need additional fuel.

- **Coordination** – Who else needs to be aware of your mission? Perhaps security forces need to know where you intend to operate and for how long. You may also need to liaise with other organizations operating in your area, to avoid duplication of effort.

- **Communications** – If you are taking radios with you, make sure that they are working, that you have spare batteries and appropriate antennae for them and that all members of your party know how to use them. Try to establish if there are likely to be any communication 'dead–spots' on your proposed route. Set procedures and timings for when you will report in to your base location during your mission.

⚡ **HAZARD**

The threat(s) – Think about what could adversely affect your ability to meet your aim. Identify dangers (climate, disease and security considerations [see Chapter 12], for example) that could affect you.

Disaster planning tools

Aspects associated with the specific planning requirements for effective post-disaster intervention are discussed elsewhere in this book. In a healthcare setting, useful planning parameters are contained in the Sphere Standards and in Médecins Sans Frontières' *Refugee Health Handbook* (see Further Reading).

● Medical preparation

There is an obvious requirement (both moral and practicable) to ensure that team members are fit and ready to deploy. There is a potential for individuals' health to deteriorate under the arduous conditions that could accompany a disaster and this could put them and others in the team at risk. It could also divert resources from the main effort of the disaster relief mission. Most good organizations will organize this for you, but **you may need to seek specialist travel medicine advice** from an appropriate clinic.

● Sources of information and advice

In addition to general health considerations, it is important to base your medical preparation on a focused health risk assessment for your deployment, consisting of the following factors:

- the destination country
- the time of year during which the deployment will take place
- the duration of the deployment
- the type of accommodation you will be using
- your role in the deployment.

Information on the destination country and its potential health implications for you as a traveller are available from a number of websites (see Table 5.2). An extremely useful and comprehensive source is the website hosted by the Health Protection Agency-funded National Travel Health Network and Centre (NaTHNaC) at www.nathnac.org. In addition to providing country-specific information, this also provides health alerts on ongoing outbreaks and incidents and advice on health protection measures, including immunizations and chemoprophylaxis.

● Packing

Health kit to pack

In addition to the antimalarial items mentioned already, you also need to consider taking with you a range of health-related equipment, to at least tide you over until you can purchase replacements. Depending upon where you're going, sunscreen may be required, although this should be obtainable locally except in the most remote locations. Similarly, pack sufficient soap, shampoo, shaving kit and toothpaste (and don't forget detergent for your clothes). Nail clippers are a good idea too.

Glasses are probably preferable to the wearing of contact lenses, which either require supplies of cleaning and disinfection fluid, or re-supply if disposables are used. Glasses are (of course) prone to damage, breakage or loss, so always pack a spare pair. Prescription sunglasses should also be considered (Ryan *et al.*, 2002).

If you require regular medication, then take sufficient to last until you can be re-supplied and, if the drugs are capable of being supplied in-country, take sufficient repeat prescriptions with you.

Table 5.2 Useful websites

Website address	Site name	Site description/remarks
www.cia.gov/library/publications/the-world-factbook	CIA World Factbook	General country-based information, including demographics, geography and topography, politics and economy. Includes health-related data
www.nathnac.org	National Travel Health Network and Centre	Country-specific travel health hazard assessment and advice on mitigation measures. Includes health alerts on outbreaks and incidents
www.fco.gov.uk/en/	Foreign and Commonwealth Office	Country-specific travel security hazard assessments and advice. Locations of UK Embassies and High Commissions. Advice on reciprocal health arrangements with UK

www.hewsweb.org	Humanitarian early warning service	Bulletin Board on expected and ongoing humanitarian emergencies
www.reliefweb.org	ReliefWeb	Bulletin Board on ongoing disasters. Includes access to maps and imagery. Useful links to other sources
www.usaid.gov/our_work/humanitarian_assistance/disaster_assistance/resources/pdf/fog_v4.pdf	US Agency for International Development (USAID) Field Operations Guide for Disaster Assessment and Response	Planning guides and practical advice for groups and individuals
www.unhcr.org/	United Nations High Commissioner for Refugees	Includes information on ongoing disasters
www.promedmail.org	Program for Monitoring of Infectious Diseases (PROMED)	Free subscription moderated bulletin board which reports on disease outbreaks and incidents worldwide
www.who.int/ith/eng/	World Health Organization International Travel and Health	Country-based advice on health threats and related mitigation measures
www.hpa.org.uk/web/HPAwebFile/HPAweb_C/1203496943523	Health Protection Agency Guidelines for malaria prevention in travellers from the UK	Country-based advice on malaria threats and appropriate preventive measures

CLINICAL CONSIDERATIONS

- Clearly, all those involved in a deployment of this nature must be checked to ensure that they are fit to fulfil their expected tasks, especially given that these are likely to be undertaken under arduous conditions. Thus, the potential impact of **any pre-existing**

medical conditions will need to be assessed and mitigated where possible.

- A **dental check-up**, followed by any necessary treatment, **is vital**, as the impact of oral emergencies can be severe.

- In addition to these general considerations, country-specific preparatory precautions are likely to be necessary. Appropriate immunizations must be given, and Yellow Fever certificates issued. These are frequently demanded at airports and border crossings into many countries (especially in Africa), as a condition of entry (Dawood, 2002).

- For malarial countries, a sufficient stock of the appropriate antimalarial drugs will need to be issued to individuals, depending upon the potential for re-supply. Those deploying will also need to **start taking their chemoprophylaxis regimen early enough** (if possible) before their expected departure date. Sufficiently robust insect repellents will need to be obtained to reduce insect vector bite-rates. **Bed-nets** (preferably treated with permethrin insecticide) should be issued, along with instructions on how to use them effectively.

PEARL OF WISDOM

In malarial countries, in addition to complying with the appropriate chemoprophylaxis regimen, the following physical precautions should also be taken:

- Cover up as much exposed skin as possible during the peak mosquito biting period (i.e. between dusk and dawn).

- Use insect repellent on the hands and face (but avoid it around the eyes and on the forehead).

- Use bed-nets at night, or use mosquito-screened accommodation.

Packing lists

While any fool can be uncomfortable on a deployment, there can be a tendency to wish to take too many unnecessary items with you. In addition to the weight involved, you must consider not taking overly expensive and attractive items with you, which could attract unwelcome attention and even encourage theft. For example, it would be sensible to take an inexpensive but reliable watch rather than one with added 'bling'.

Packing considerations

The requirements for your personal equipment will be driven by a number of factors:

- the climate of the destination country
- the type of accommodation you will be living in
- the expected duration of the deployment
- your access to transport in-country
- the maximum baggage allowance granted

PEARL OF WISDOM

- Travel as light as possible. Only take what you can carry yourself.
- Pack your belongings in a robust rucksack.
- Ensure that you can secure your belongings. Lockable security nets are now readily available to protect rucksacks.
- Take smaller day-sacks for short-term use, so that you don't need to take all your belongings with you all the time.

- the possibilities for re-supply (either in-country or from home)
- your task(s) during the deployment.

Personal equipment

Once you have established the climate you're going to be working in and how you will be accommodated, you can start to decide what you need to pack. Essentially, consider:

- **How will you be sleeping?** Do you need a sleeping bag alone, or a full sleeping system with insulation mat and a weatherproof cover?
- **How will you be fed?** As a minimum, you should pack knife, fork and spoon and a mug, although you might need to take utensils and a means of cooking food *in extremis*.
- **How will you be supplied with drinking water?** Although the provision of safe water is probably best organized communally, it may be prudent to take your own personal water purifier which has the capability of both filtering and disinfecting a contaminated supply.
- **What clothing will you require?** Basic requirements are that this should be hard-wearing, easy to wash using very basic facilities and looking as non-military as possible. The latter is extremely important in complex emergencies and areas of conflict, where it is best not to be confused as having any military connections or role. To protect yourself from the elements, you may need to take several layers of clothing, with the outer one being waterproof. Don't forget appropriate headwear such as a sun hat (for hot climates) or a thermal hat (for cold climates).
- **What footwear do you need?** Lightweight but robust boots are ideal, **provided they have been well broken in first**. It is also well worth packing sandals ('flip-flops' are ideal).
- **What other items do you think you might need or want** during your deployment? A torch (preferably a head torch) is essential. A cheap digital camera is useful. Do not

expect to be working all of the time, so take paperbacks with you (these can be swapped with other members of your team, and left behind when you come home), although check what is and is not considered acceptable in the destination country. Similarly, a personal stereo will be a useful recreational distraction when off duty, as will playing cards and travel versions of board games. To maintain links with home and to lessen potential feelings of isolation, a battery-operated multi-band radio, capable of picking up the BBC World Service is worth packing. If at all possible, try to choose electrical appliances that use the same types and sizes of battery, as this will ease potential problems with re-supply. In addition to recreational items, try to make space for a multi-tool and a sewing kit for running repairs on clothes (Ryan *et al.*, 2002).

HAZARD

Do you need to take any role-specific items of equipment? Wherever possible, these should be transported under communal arrangements, rather than being carried by individuals, especially if they include drugs and sharps, the personal carriage of which in some countries is considered illegal.

The packing process

Once you have assembled all of your personal kit, pack essentials for the journey (making allowances for delays in transit) into a day-sack and keep this with you as cabin baggage. Measure and weigh it to ensure it meets current baggage allowances.

Pack everything else into your main bag, weigh it, lock it and label it.

● Finance

Finance to cover the mission of your intended deployment should be provided by your employing agency. You will, however, need to make arrangements to cover incidentals and personal expenses.

Where possible, take travellers' cheques in sterling or US dollars, but also take some cash, especially in small denomination notes. It is probably best to take local currency for this (if available), although US dollars may be an alternative. You need to check, however, that the use of foreign currency is not considered illegal in the country in which you will be working. Especially, **be wary of attempting to change your money into local currency anywhere other than in a recognized bank or bureau de change**.

Find out from your employing agency if and how they will be paying you for the duration of the deployment and make arrangements as necessary from home to send you further travellers' cheques or money orders.

● Insurance

You will need to **consider a range of insurance** to cover your intended deployment (Ryan *et al.*, 2002):

- Insurance for the **personal equipment and effects** that you are taking with you. As discussed previously, such items need to be kept to a minimum and you should take sensible precautions against damage or theft (such as not openly displaying potentially attractive or valuable effects).
- Insurance against **death or personal injury**.
- Insurance to cover **medical treatment** and possible repatriation to the United Kingdom. There are reciprocal health arrangements between a number of countries (within the European Union, for example), where some treatment and even hospitalization may be provided free or at reduced cost. Even under such circumstances, free

treatment will be offered only on proof of nationality. Within the EU, you will need to possess a European Health Insurance Card, which can be applied for on-line at: www.nhs.uk/EHIC/Pages/Applyingandrenewing.aspx

- Advice is available from the Foreign and Commonwealth Office (www.fco.gov.uk) on which countries have reciprocal arrangements for treatment of United Kingdom nationals. It also provides useful advice on insurance to cover repatriation to home should you be involved in an accident or become ill. **Do not underestimate the potential costs involved in repatriation** under these circumstances.
- Although your employing agency may organize all of the above for you, **you must check**.

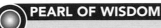

PEARL OF WISDOM

- Always ensure that the level of cover provided under your insurance policies is appropriate for your personal needs and requirements.
- Always ensure that your insurers are aware of the type of work that you will be undertaking.

● Readjustment on return

Chapter 9 of this book provides definitive advice on identifying and coping with mental health issues associated with aid work. This chapter will therefore cover general tips to help you, your family, colleagues and friends cope with readjusting to 'normal' life after returning from a deployment.

What to expect

You will probably have been entirely focused on your mission; perhaps for a significant period of time. Although you may well have tried to communicate to your friends and family what you have seen and done by letter, phone or e-mail during the deployment, you will have to accept that they will not really understand your experience (especially if you have censored your messages, in an attempt to spare them from concern about your safety and well-being). You will undoubtedly want to go home, but your expectations may be a bit over-blown. Take time to realistically prepare; wind down and try to rehearse in your mind what went right, what went wrong and prepare for the inevitable question 'So how was it, then?' (Ryan *et al.*, 2002).

When you return, people (even those close to you) will not understand (how could they?) what you have experienced and you might find this attitude annoying. In addition, never forget that things ('normal' things) have continued to happen to them. If you have been away for several months, even close family members will have developed or coped in their own way. This can be especially difficult if you have small children. Be prepared to be angry, irritable (because people don't understand your experience), guilty (that you feel that you've come home too soon) and frustrated (because your experience has changed you).

What to do

- Document what you've done and write reports.
- Take pictures while you are deployed to help people understand your experience.
- Keep in contact with those you deployed with; they are probably going through the same experience that you are.
- Try to feel proud about your achievements, both personally and as part of your team.
- **If you are concerned, seek professional support.**

Summary

- Becoming involved in disaster relief interventions can be rewarding, but you should only do so after due consideration.
- Be prepared to work as part of a team... if you are not a team player then this type of work is probably not for you.

- Reduce the risks to you, your team colleagues and your mission by appropriate planning.
- Protect your health during deployment by taking appropriate measures following a comprehensive health risk assessment. If necessary consult a travel medicine professional.
- Only take what personal and technical equipment you need, based on your plan.
- Make suitable arrangements for personal finance and ensure that you and your kit are appropriately insured.
- Prepare yourself for making the necessary adjustments back to 'normal' life. Do not expect too much, and seek specialist professional advice if necessary.

REFERENCES AND FURTHER READING

References

Adair J. *The Skills of Leadership*. Gower, Aldershot, 1984.

Dawood R. *Travellers' Health: how to stay healthy abroad*. Oxford: Oxford University Press, 2002.

Handy S. *Understanding Voluntary Organizations*. Penguin, London, New York, Victoria, Ontario and Wellington, 1988.

Hodgkinson P and Stewart M. *Coping with Catastrophe. A handbook of disaster management*. Routledge, London and New York, 1991.

Lloyd Roberts D. *Staying Alive – safety and security guidelines for humanitarian volunteers*. Geneva: International Committee of the Red Cross, 2005.

Ryan J, Mahoney P, Greaves I and Bowyer G. (eds) *Conflict and Catastrophe Medicine – a practical guide*. Springer, London, 2002.

Further reading

Hanquet A. (ed.) *Refugee Health – an approach to emergency situations*. Macmillan, London, 1997.

McConnan I. (ed.) *The Sphere Project Humanitarian Charter and Minimum Standards in Disaster Response*. Oxfam Publishing, Oxford, 2000.

6 Medicine in the field

Tim O'Dempsey

● Introduction

Tropical and infectious diseases are the leading causes of death and disability among vulnerable populations in low-income countries. In terms of risk of exposure and impact of natural disasters and complex humanitarian emergencies, the burden of disease is greatest among poor populations that have the least coping capacity.

Inadequate water and sanitation and poor environmental and housing conditions favour the transmission of pathogens that are spread by the faeco-oral route, droplet, direct contact and vectors. The relative importance of specific pathogens may vary depending on geographical and environmental conditions. Knowing what is likely to be out there is key to effective clinical practice in these situations.

Displacement may expose individuals of all ages to previously unencountered infectious diseases. Such conditions favour the occurrence of epidemics that may rapidly involve large numbers of susceptible individuals and overwhelm available health services.

Dislocation from and disruption of family and community networks further increases vulnerability to exploitation and poses additional risk of HIV and other sexually transmitted

PEARL OF WISDOM

Cultural determinants of healthcare-seeking behaviour are of great importance, particularly among traditional peoples that hitherto may have had few or no better alternatives in the provision for their health needs.

infections. Such risks are compounded in situations of conflict that are often associated with high levels of sexual violence.

Lack of availability, accessibility, affordability and adequacy of health services means that people often present late to mainstream services having previously sought treatment from **sources including traditional healers, local shops and pharmacies, market traders and drug peddlers**.

HAZARD

Local medicines that are available may be counterfeit, substandard or may have been tampered with.

Recommended immunizations may have been unavailable or ineffective due to deficiencies in the cold chain. Measles can cause devastating epidemics in these circumstances with severe acute complications, high case fatality rates or long-term complications such as blindness occurring in children who are vitamin A deficient or otherwise malnourished. Nutritional status may be poor due to food insecurity and compounded by the vicious cycle of infection, impaired immunity, inadequate intake and malnutrition.

An awareness of these complexities is essential for clinical work in austere environments. We are frequently faced with individuals who present late in the course of an illness, who may have multiple underlying health problems and who, prior to presentation, may have received a variety of treatments of varying efficacy or toxicity.

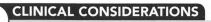

CLINICAL CONSIDERATIONS

- **An empathic understanding of culture and context is a prerequisite** for the successful diagnosis and management of clinical problems.
- **We must rely on our skills in history taking and clinical examination**, overcoming language and communication barriers. We may have limited or no laboratory and other diagnostic facilities. Our restricted range of drugs and other therapeutic resources can be compromised by unreliable logistics, insecurity, seasonal and other threats. In an unselected caseload more than half of our patients are likely to be children. Therefore, it is important to have good clinical knowledge and experience of paediatrics. We are unlikely to have ready access to highly experienced colleagues to whom we can turn for advice when faced with difficult clinical problems.
- **We must be prepared to assume the roles** of physician, paediatrician, obstetrician, surgeon, psychiatrist, epidemiologist, public health specialist, pathologist and, sometimes, dentist.

Some of the most important tropical infectious diseases are listed in Table 6.1. Clearly it is impossible to discuss all of these in detail within a brief chapter. Readers are referred to the documents listed under Further Reading at the end of the chapter, most of which are freely available as pdf files.

In this chapter we will use a series of clinical scenarios to illustrate some of the commonest clinical presentations of infectious diseases likely to be encountered in low-resource settings.

Although tuberculosis and HIV infections are likely to be highly prevalent and important among poor people affected

Table 6.1 Important infectious diseases in the tropics

Parasitic infections:
Malaria
African trypanosomiasis
American trypanosomiasis
Leishmaniasis (visceral/cutaneous/mucocutaneous)
Schistosomiasis and other flukes
Lymphatic filariasis, onchocerciasis, loa loa, Guinea worm
Gut protozoa (e.g. amoebiasis, giardiasis, cryptosporidia, microsporidia, etc.)
Soil-transmitted helminths (e.g. roundworm, hookworm, strongyloides, trichuris, etc.)
Cestodes (e.g. tapeworms, cysticercosis, hydatidosis)

Other infectious diseases of importance in the tropics:
Acute respiratory infections
Measles and other Expanded Programme on Immunization (EPI) vaccine preventable infections
Meningitis
Tuberculosis
Leprosy
Brucellosis
Cholera, dysentery, other diarrhoeal diseases
Typhoid and non-typhoid salmonella infections
Typhus
Relapsing fever
Plague
Anthrax
Melioidosis
Spirochaetoses
Leptospirosis
Hepatitis
Sexually transmitted infections (STIs), HIV
Arboviruses
Viral haemorrhagic fevers
Rabies
Fungal infections

by conflict and catastrophe, specific management of these problems are not discussed in detail in this chapter. Their management is relatively complex and requires prolonged and reliable organizational and logistical support for the implementation of treatment protocols that ideally should comply with national policy.

In poor countries, adults with HIV infection are more likely to die because of pneumococcal, salmonella or other common 'community acquired' infections than because of the HIV associated 'opportunistic' infections that emerge when patients develop low CD4 counts in more affluent settings.

Tuberculosis has a plethora of acute and chronic clinical presentations and should be considered in the differential diagnosis of almost all other infectious diseases in the tropics. TB may present clinically when an individual becomes debilitated by other infection, particularly HIV, following severe measles or associated with malnutrition and should always be considered in such patients if they are failing to respond to nutritional support and treatment of other infections.

Conditions of poor hygiene and sanitation are associated with a high prevalence of protozoal infections (e.g. amoebiasis, giardiasis, cryptosporidiosis, microsporidiosis) and helminthic infections (e.g. roundworm, hookworm, strongyloides, trichuris, schistosomiasis and other flukes). Migrating helminths can cause wheeze, urticarial rashes and eosinophilia.

Multiple parasitic infections are common. Infected individuals may present with acute or chronic symptoms that are caused by a specific parasite, may present with other illnesses but be debilitated by co-infection with these parasites, or may be asymptomatic. Immunosuppression may result in severe illness and particular care should be taken to exclude or treat for amoebiasis and strongyloidiasis in patients prior to treatment with immunosuppressive drugs, including steroids. A 'watching brief' should also be maintained for reactivation of TB in patients who are immunosuppressed.

Albendazole or mebendazole are effective for treating roundworm, hookworm and trichuris. Ivermectin should be used for strongyloides. Metronidazole is effective in amoebiasis and giardiasis. Albendazole is also useful for microsporidiosis.

Praziquantel is used for treating schistosomiasis, other flukes and cestode infections with the exception of *Fasciola hepatica* and *F. gigantica* for which triclabendazole is recommended.

Nitazoxanide is a relatively new drug that is effective in the treatment of a wide range of gastrointestinal parasites including *Entamoebal histolytica*, *Giardia intestinalis (G. lamblia)*, *Cyclospora cayetanensis*, *Cryptosporidium parvum*, *Enterocytozoon bieneusi*, *Ascaris lumbricoides*, *Strongyloides stercoralis*, *Trichuris trichiura*, *Enterobius vermicularis*, *Taenia saginata*, *Hymenolepis nana* and *Fasciola hepatica*. In immunocompetent patients, a 3-day course of oral nitazoxanide is usually recommended in the following doses:

- adults and children over 12 years, 500 mg b.d.
- children aged 4–11 years, 200 mg b.d.
- children aged 1–3 years, 100 mg b.d.

Nitazoxanide is becoming the drug of choice for HIV-related cryptosporidiosis and, because of its broad spectrum of activity, may have a role in the 'blind' treatment of persistent diarrhoea in circumstances where diagnostic facilities are limited or absent.

● Syndromic management of common clinical problems

The Integrated Management of Childhood Illness (IMCI) developed by WHO provides a useful approach to the diagnosis and management of common childhood infectious and other diseases in resource-limited settings, particularly where laboratory facilities are unavailable.

Designed for use by health workers with limited clinical training, IMCI guidelines provide clear diagnostic and management pathways for children presenting with fever, cough or difficulty breathing, diarrhoea, ear problems, malnutrition and anaemia. Specific guidelines are also included for assessing and managing children with 'danger signs' that may indicate severe illness. Additional guidelines are available for young infants <2 months and for management of childhood illnesses in settings with a high HIV seroprevalence. A similar approach is used in WHO's Integrated Management of Adolescent and Adult Illness (IMAI).

● Public health approach to communicable disease control in emergencies

In emergency situations with large numbers of vulnerable, debilitated persons living in crowded conditions with poor standards of hygiene, sanitation and shelter, it is essential to establish public health systems for the control of communicable diseases. This involves three areas for action:

1. **Rapid assessment** – should include identification of the main communicable disease threats, especially those with epidemic potential, in the host country, the country of origin of displaced persons and the areas through which they may have passed. Public health priorities should be identified and health coordination mechanisms established through the lead agency for health.

2. **Prevention of communicable diseases** – requires care in site selection and planning, including adequate water and sanitation facilities and vector control measures. Essential nutritional requirements must be met. Immunization

programmes must be established as soon as possible, particularly for prevention of measles. Basic clinical and laboratory services must also be established.

3. **Surveillance and early warning systems** – Surveillance is the ongoing systematic collection, analysis and interpretation of data in order to plan, implement and evaluate public health interventions. Minimum data sets, case definitions, recording and reporting systems must be agreed for monitoring disease trends and to ensure that outbreaks are detected, reported and investigated early.

The basic steps in investigating an outbreak are summarized in the Learning Points box below. This approach should be applied to all communicable diseases with epidemic potential.

LEARNING POINTS

Basic steps in managing an outbreak

- Verify the existence of an outbreak – has the epidemic threshold been exceeded?
- Confirm diagnosis – obtain appropriate samples for laboratory tests.
- Implement immediate control measures if necessary.
- Develop a case definition.
- Identify cases: population at risk – calculate attack rate.
- Follow up cases and contacts.
- Describe the outbreak – person, place, time (Who? What? When? Where? Why? How?)
- Formulate hypotheses for pathogen, source, transmission.
- Test hypotheses – conduct further investigations and epidemiological studies.
- Analyse and communicate findings.
- Plan additional studies – involve external agencies if necessary.

- Develop and implement control measures – treat cases, prevent transmission.
- Evaluate preparedness, surveillance, response and outcomes.
- Write and circulate report and recommendations concerning the outbreak.

● Case studies

The following case studies illustrate five of the most important acute clinical tropical and infectious disease problems that are likely to be encountered in low resource settings, often in the context of epidemics.

CASE STUDY 1

Fever and coma in an African child

Situation: Rural lowland East Africa, rainy season. 50 miles from the nearest in-patient facility. Roads are dreadful and rivers liable to flood. You are the medical doctor leading a small mobile clinic team (one midwife, one junior nurse, one driver).

After a bumpy and muddy four hour journey in your four-wheel-drive vehicle you reach the clinic location. It is 11.00 hours. Clustered beneath some trees a crowd of 200–300 people awaits the clinic. You are unloading your equipment when a distressed woman carrying a baby rushes up to you. Your driver interprets.

The baby is about 12 months old. He was well until yesterday morning when he developed high fever, watery diarrhoea, vomiting and was initially refusing, later unable, to feed. As the day went on he became weaker. During the night he had a series of generalized convulsions. His mother was unable to wake him this morning and has walked 10 miles to the mobile clinic. He has not been given any medicine so far.

On rapid initial examination of the baby you note the following:

- deeply unconscious, unresponsive to pain, Blantyre coma score < 3 (see box below);
- sunken eyes, reduced skin turgor, sunken anterior fontanelle;
- cold peripheries, capillary refill > 2 seconds, weak rapid pulse;
- pale conjunctiva, mucous membranes, palmar creases, nail beds;
- deep, sighing respirations; respiratory rate 30 breaths/min;
- nutritional status good;
- no rash.

What are you going to do?

CLINICAL CONSIDERATIONS

The Blantyre coma scale is a modification of the Glasgow coma scale suitable for use in young children

Response	Findings	Score
Best motor response	Localizes to painful stimulus	2
	Withdraws limb from painful stimulus	1
	No response or inappropriate response	0
Best verbal response	Vocalizes appropriately with painful stimulus	2
	Moan or abnormal cry with painful stimulus	1
	No vocal response to painful stimulus	0
Eye movement	Watches or follows (e.g. mother's face)	1
	Fails to watch or follow	0

Blantyre coma score = best motor response + best verbal response + eye movement.
Interpretation: Abnormal < 5; Unrousable coma < 3.

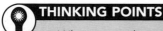

THINKING POINTS

- What immediate management is required?
- What is our working differential diagnosis?
- What on-going management is required?

Immediate management

Explain to the mother what you are doing and why. She will be very anxious and frightened. This child is at significant risk of dying. The mother is unlikely to be familiar with modern medical practice and her perception of cause and effect may be such that, if the child dies, she may believe that what you have done has caused or contributed to the child's death, for example taking blood, putting up a drip and so on.

Resuscitation

- **ABC** – Ensure the airway is clear and the child is breathing.
- **Circulation** – Establish intravenous (iv) or intraosseous (io) access.

PEARL OF WISDOM

It may be difficult to establish iv access – make sure that you are familiar with and prepared to insert an intraosseous line.

- **Treat for shock:** 20 ml/kg normal saline iv/io. Repeat once if necessary.
- Appropriate **volume resuscitation** is also important in correcting the metabolic acidosis that commonly complicates severe malaria or sepsis.
- **DEFG, Don't Ever Forget Glucose** – Hypoglycaemia may complicate severe malaria and other serious infections in children. Exclude or treat empirically for hypoglycaemia: 5 ml/kg of 10 per cent dextrose. This is given in addition to the 20 ml/kg of normal saline for shock.

- 'Prophylactic' anticonvulsants are not routinely recommended despite the history of convulsions. However, if the child has a convulsion, give **rectal diazepam** 0.5 mg/kg. If the convulsion continues, repeat after 10 min. (Diazepam may also be given very slowly iv but beware of respiratory depression.)
- If there is no response after a second dose of diazepam give **rectal paraldehyde** 0.3–0.4 ml/kg. Paraldehyde may also be given im **(but NOT iv)**. Paraldehyde is excellent for controlling acute convulsions. Paraldehyde 'melts' plastic, but may be administered using a plastic syringe, provided it is given immediately after drawing up the dose.

Working differential diagnosis

1. Severe malaria.
2. Meningitis/septicaemia.

The differential diagnosis is more extensive than indicated in our working diagnosis. However, this working diagnosis enables us to take a systematic and comprehensive approach to clinical management that would be appropriate in this scenario.

The clinical presentation points to severe malaria with complications including cerebral malaria, anaemia, metabolic acidosis and hypoglycaemia (Table 6.2).

A similar presentation may occur in meningitis, sepsis or other overwhelming infection. The possibility of an underlying condition that may predispose the child to severe infection, such as HIV infection or sickle cell disease, should also be considered as should the possibility of metabolic disease or complications due to the use of traditional or other medications.

Ongoing management

Severe malaria

If available, use a Rapid Diagnostic Test (RDT) for malaria. If an RDT is not available, make a thick blood film for later

Table 6.2 Manifestations of severe malaria

Manifestations of cerebral malaria (defined as unrousable coma not attributable to any other cause in a patient with *P. falciparum* malaria):

Generalized convulsions

Severe anaemia

Hypoglycaemia

Metabolic acidosis with respiratory distress

Hyperpyrexia (core temperature $>42°C$)

Hyperparasitaemia (>2 per cent RBCs infected if 'non-immune')

Fluid and electrolyte disturbances

Acute renal failure

Haemoglobinuria

Acute pulmonary oedema/adult respiratory distress (ARDS)

Circulatory collapse, shock, Gram-negative septicaemia ('algid malaria')

Abnormal bleeding (including disseminated intravascular coagulation [DIC])

Jaundice, hepatic dysfunction

Splenic rupture.

Important: These severe manifestations can occur singly or, more commonly, in combination in the same patient.

examination when laboratory facilities become available. Cover the slide to prevent flies feasting on the blood or there will be nothing left on the slide to stain!

Treat empirically for severe malaria. Where available and appropriate, follow national guidelines for management of malaria. These should be kept up to date and should reflect current information concerning drug resistance.

In this scenario the following antimalarial drugs should be considered for initial management:

First choice for severe malaria: **artesunate**.

- Artesunate iv/io/im/pr. This is a rapidly acting antimalarial that can be administered by a variety of routes:
  - iv/im 2.4 mg/kg initially, followed by 1.2 mg/kg iv or im after 12 hours, then daily for a minimum of 3 days until

the child can take oral treatment of another effective antimalarial.

- Rectal artesunate suppositories (10 mg/kg), if available, can provide an effective way for village health workers with limited training and resources to initiate treatment for severe malaria prior to referral for further management.

Complete treatment in severe malaria following parenteral artesunate or artemether administration by giving a full course of artemisinin-based combination therapy (ACT) for example, artemether-lumefantrine, or artesunate + amodiaquine, or oral quinine to complete 7 days of treatment. If available and affordable, quinine should be combined with clindamycin.

Second choice for severe malaria: **quinine.**

If artesunate is not available give quinine (most commonly available as quinine dihydrochloride). An initial loading dose of quinine 20 mg/kg in 5 ml/kg of 5 per cent dextrose by iv infusion over 4 hours, is followed by maintenance infusions of 10 mg/kg in 5 ml/kg of 5 per cent dextrose over 4 hours every 8 hours until the child is able to take oral treatment.

However, in the circumstances described, iv quinine may not be advisable: who will monitor the infusion? You and your team have 200–300 other patients to manage. If the infusion cannot be carefully monitored, it may be safer to give the quinine im. Remember quinine may induce hypoglycaemia. Therefore, if possible, monitor blood glucose if quinine is used.

Severe malaria may also be complicated by Gram-negative septicaemia. This leads us to the next step in our working diagnosis.

Meningitis/sepsis
- Can we confidently exclude meningitis or septicaemia? If not, give appropriate antibiotics in addition to the antimalarial treatment.

- The commonest causes of meningitis in this age group are pneumococcal, meningococcal and *Haemophilus influenzae* type B.
- Common causes of septicaemia include the above plus *Staphylococcus aureus*, non-typhoid salmonella and other Gram-negative organisms.

The choice of antibiotic will be based on the likely organisms and their likely antibiotic sensitivity. If available, ceftriaxone would be a reasonable first-line choice of antibiotic in these circumstances. However, chloramphenicol is more likely to be available and would usually be effective in covering the likely range of possible bacterial pathogens.

Supportive management

Maintenance fluids
Maintenance iv fluids pose a similar monitoring problem to those discussed above. Therefore, oral rehydration solution via a nasogastric tube may be necessary for maintenance fluids and to reduce further risk of hypoglycaemia.

Temperature
Fever is an appropriate physiological response to infection. On balance, arguments against treating fever outweigh those in favour. However, active management of fever is indicated for hyperpyrexia or for children who are seriously ill as in this case, where high fever may further compromise the metabolic state. If it is available give paracetamol rectally or via a nasogastric tube. Active cooling is recommended in cases of hyperpyrexia. Tepid sponging, although widely practised, should not be encouraged.

Further management
When you have addressed the issues above, one further dilemma remains: Should we transfer this child to hospital immediately or wait until we have finished our clinic?

The key question is: What additional life-saving measures are available only in the hospital?

The one remaining specific measure that may be critical for this child's survival and that is unlikely to be possible in the field, is a blood transfusion. **Blood transfusion is recommended for children with severe malaria associated with acute anaemia where Hb < 5 g/100 ml.**

The final decision to transfer also requires consideration of the following:

- How long will the trip to the hospital take?
- How long will it take for the vehicle to return?
- How sure can we be about travel times given the state of the roads and unpredictable weather-related events, for example, rivers in flood?
- Will the child survive the journey?
- Will blood be available?
- Do we need to send/bring a relative with the child to donate blood?
- Which member of your team should accompany the child?
- Do we pack up the clinic now or wait for the vehicle to return?
- What do we do about the other patients?

Conclusion

The case study discussed above will be encountered on a daily basis in regions endemic for *Plasmodium falciparum*. In reality, mobile clinic teams rarely include a doctor. The approach we have outlined provides an action plan for the management of any child presenting with severe malaria or sepsis, which can be implemented by anyone on the team with appropriate clinical training.

Rapid onset of severe diarrhoea and dehydration in an adult plus the fact that adults as well as children are affected in the community is highly suggestive of a **cholera epidemic**.

In this situation we need to think about management of affected individuals and prevention of infection in those at risk. A cholera epidemic can place a severe strain on all resources (staff, inpatient and outpatient facilities, fluids, antibiotics, etc.). Successful management depends on careful preparedness and contingency planning, effective communication and robust logistical support.

Management of individual patients

Start with ABC principles.

Fluids

Fluid replacement and maintenance is the key to managing cases of cholera (Table 6.3). An adult may lose 500–1000 ml/hour.

Table 6.3 Management of dehydration associated with diarrhoeal diseases

Dehydration	Management of dehydration	
	Signs	Treatment
Severe	Lethargic, unconscious, floppy, very sunken eyes, very poor skin turgor, very dry mouth, drinks poorly or unable to drink	iv therapy (Ringer lactate) 100 ml/kg over 3–6 h Age < 1 yr: 30 ml/kg over 60 min then: 70 ml/kg over 5 h Age > 1 yr: 30 ml/kg over 30 min then: 70 ml/kg over 2.5 h +ORS
Mild–moderate	Restless and irritable, sunken eyes, poor skin turgor, dry mouth, thirsty, drinks eagerly	ORS 75 ml/kg over 4 h plus very close surveillance
None	None of the above signs	ORS at home Give ORS as soon as diarrhoea starts Give ORS after each loose stool

ORS, oral rehydration solution.

Home-made oral rehydration solution (ORS)

If ORS packets are unavailable, simple ORS can be prepared by mixing the following ingredients:

- One level teaspoon of salt.
- Eight level teaspoons of sugar.
- One litre of clean water.

Addition of half a cup of freshly squeezed orange juice or mixing in some banana will provide a source of potassium.

Rice and other cereal-based ORS solutions can also be used. Reduced osmolarity ORS is now preferred in the management of diarrhoea although, patients with cholera may develop hyponatraemia.

Chlorpromazine, acting as an antisecretory agent, is occasionally used as an adjunct to fluid management.

Antibiotics

Antibiotics shorten the period of diarrhoea and reduce fluid loss. Antibiotic use is usually restricted to severe cases. Antibiotic resistance is common and choice will depend on knowledge of local sensitivities. Ciprofloxacin, doxycycline, co-trimoxazole or erythromycin may be suitable.

Infection control measures

Cholera is highly infectious. If possible, cases should be managed in a specific cholera isolation and treatment facility (ward, tent, isolation room as appropriate according to number of cases and resources available). Faecal material and vomit must be properly disinfected and disposed of. Ideally, severe cases should be managed on a 'cholera cot', a waterproof covered mattress with a central hole beneath which is placed a bucket for collection of faeces. Visiting should be restricted to one carer who should be briefed on the importance of personal hygiene, particularly handwashing, in minimizing risk of transmission.

Prophylactic antibiotics are not recommended for medical staff or other contacts. The emphasis should be on personal hygiene and hand washing. Oral cholera vaccine is recommended for medical staff working in at-risk situations.

Confirm the diagnosis

Diagnosis is presumptive in epidemics. Cases should be managed as though they have cholera whilst steps are taken to confirm a possible epidemic. Dark field microscopy of faecal material may reveal darting vibrios. Rectal swabs/ faeces are transported in alkaline peptone water or Cary Blair medium. Confirmation is by culture of stool/rectal swab on thiosulphate citrate bile salts sucrose (TCBS) agar. Specimens should be sent to a reference laboratory for biotyping and serotyping. Antibiotic sensitivity tests should be performed on a sample of isolates. A number of rapid diagnostic tests for cholera have recently become available, for example Cholera SMART™ (Sensitive Membrane Antigen Rapid Test), which has been used in the field by Médecins Sans Frontières (MSF).

L **LEARNING POINT**

Cholera is an internationally notifiable disease.

Public health measures

Apply the principles of outbreak investigation (see Learning points box on steps in managing an outbreak on pp. 132–3).

One suspected case of cholera, particularly in situations involving displaced populations or damaged water/sanitation infrastructure, should prompt immediate action. Specifying a case definition is important for surveillance purposes. Case definitions may vary between organizations.

Examples of case definitions for cholera

MSF cholera case definition

Any patient developing rapid onset severe watery diarrhoea (usually with vomiting), resulting in severe dehydration.

WHO cholera case definitions

- In an area in which cholera is not known to be present, any patient ⩾ 5 years who develops severe dehydration or dies from acute watery diarrhoea.
- In an area in which there is a cholera outbreak, any patient ⩾ 5 years who develops acute watery diarrhoea, with or without vomiting.

All organizations that are engaged in cholera surveillance in a particular area should use the same case definition.

The following immediate control measures should be undertaken:

- **Prompt diagnosis** and appropriate treatment of patients.
- Establish **peripheral ORS stations** so that people have early access to fluids.
- Establish **treatment centres** with nursing precautions appropriate for enteric pathogens.

- Conduct **health education programmes** on hygiene, disinfection and sanitation measures with simple messages on safe water, safe food and handwashing with soap and clean water.

Cholera deaths

The case fatality rate should be < 2 per cent among patients requiring admission.

⚡ HAZARD

Dead bodies after cholera pose a significant public health risk and great care must be taken in the handling and disposal of the dead. Funerals should be held quickly and near the place of death. Those who prepare the body for burial must be meticulous about handwashing and if possible wear gloves and an apron. A mask is also recommended, principally to reduce the likelihood of faeco-oral contamination. The corpse should be disinfected with a 2 per cent chlorine solution and the mouth and anus filled with chlorine-soaked cotton wool. The intestines should not be emptied. The head should be bandaged so that the mouth remains shut. The corpse should be wrapped and corpse-carriers should wear gloves. Funeral feasts should be discouraged or banned.

Oral cholera vaccine

Oral cholera vaccine may have a role in preventing spread in the community. WHO recommend a three-step process when considering mass immunization with oral cholera vaccine:

- Assess risk of a cholera outbreak.
- Assess whether key public health priorities are or can be implemented in a timely manner and assess the capacity to respond to a possible outbreak.
- Assess the feasibility of an immunization campaign.

The vaccine currently recommended consists of killed *Vibrio cholerae 01* plus recombinant cholera B subunit (WC/rBS vaccine). Two oral doses (three doses if age 2–6 years) are recommended 10–14 days apart, avoiding food for 1 hour before and after each dose. Protection commences about 10 days after the second dose. A booster is required after 2 years (or after 6 months for children aged 2–6 years). Protective efficacy in adults is 85–90 per cent after 6 months falling to 62 per cent at 1 year in cholera-endemic regions. There is also evidence of a herd immunity effect.

CASE STUDY 3

An outbreak of dysentery in South America

Situation – Rural Bolivia. Three members of a family – mother, father and 4-year-old boy, present to your clinic with the following complaints:

- Mother – diarrhoea containing blood and abdominal cramps worsening over the past 4 days.
- Father – diarrhoea containing blood and abdominal cramps worsening over the past 2 days.
- Boy – ill for the past 3 days – diarrhoea initially watery, days now complaining of abdominal cramps, diarrhoea with blood and fever.

Several other families in the village have had similar symptoms over the past week. In the previous 4 weeks only three cases of diarrhoea with blood were recorded in the clinic register.

What are you going to do?

In this context, diarrhoea with visible blood indicates dysentery. The main differential is between bacillary and amoebic dysentery. In the case above, bacillary dysentery is more likely. The principle clues are the symptoms of abdominal cramps and fever both of which tend to be comparatively early symptoms in shigellosis. The commonest cause of epidemic dysentery in developing countries is *Shigella dysenteriae* type 1.

Simple microscopy may solve this diagnostic problem – Amoebic dysentery, caused by *Entamoeba histolytica,* can be diagnosed by examining a fresh stool specimen for motile amoebic trophozoites characterized by the presence of ingested red blood cells (RBCs) within the cytoplasm. The presence of amoebic cysts is not diagnostic of amoebic dysentery as *E. histolytica* cysts are identical to cysts of *Entamoeba dispar*, which is non-pathogenic. Similarly, non-pathogenic amoebic trophozoites that do not contain RBCs may be seen in patients with diarrhoea due to any cause. Amoebic trophozoites without ingested RBCs are not diagnostic of amoebic dysentery.

The fact that there has been **an unexpected increase in the number of cases implies an epidemic**. Therefore management must be directed at identifying the causative organism, establishing antibiotic sensitivities, managing individual cases and managing the epidemic.

Diagnosis should be confirmed by culture of a rectal swab, transported in buffered 30 per cent glycerol saline. Multi-drug resistant strains are widespread, therefore antibiotic sensitivity testing is essential at an early stage in an outbreak.

Individual case management

Fluids
Principles of fluid management for dysentery and other diarrhoeal diseases are similar to those indicated previously for cholera.

Antibiotics (Table 6.4)
Mild cases of shigellosis should not normally require antibiotics. Antibiotics are indicated for more severe cases and in situations of crowding where standards of hygiene and sanitation are poor. Ciprofloxacin is a reasonable choice for

Table 6.4 Antimicrobials for treatment of shigellosis

Antimicrobial	Treatment schedule	
	Children	Adults
Ciprofloxacin (first choice)	15 mg/kg 2 times per day for 3 days, orally	500 mg 2 times per day for 3 days, orally
Pivmecillinam	20 mg/kg 4 times per day for 5 days, orally	100 mg 4 times per day for 5 days, orally
Ceftriaxone	50–100 mg/kg once a day im for 2 to 5 days	–
Azithromycin	6–20 mg/kg once a day for 1 to 5 days, orally	1–1.5 g once a day for 1 to 5 days, orally

Modified from WHO, 2005.

empiric treatment. Note that haemolytic uraemic syndrome (HUS) complicates about 13 per cent of hospitalized cases of *Shigella dysenteriae* type 1. The risk of HUS is increased in enterohaemorrhagic *Escherichia coli* infections, for example *E. coli* 0157, when treated with antibiotics. Given that *Shigella* is really an *E. coli*, the risk:benefit ratio of using antibiotics needs to be carefully weighed.

Other treatment

- **Zinc** – supplementation in children aged less than 5 years reduces the frequency, severity and persistence of diarrhoea (including dysentery).
- **Vitamin A** – also reduces severity of episodes of diarrhoea (including dysentery).

Public health measures

These are similar to those indicated for cholera, however, the risks associated with handling of corpses are less and the stringent regulations indicated for cholera are not usually necessary. There are no effective vaccines available for *Shigella*.

The presentation above is consistent with **acute meningitis**. In the absence of contraindications, the investigation of choice is lumbar puncture (LP).

THINKING POINTS

Cerebrospinal fluid (CSF) examination where there is no laboratory

A great deal of information can be obtained by LP even without sophisticated laboratory facilities. Cloudy CSF with a short history would be highly suggestive of bacterial meningitis. If the CSF looks clear on inspection, reagent strips for testing urine are a good substitute for a biochemistry laboratory and can be used to indicate whether there is raised protein, low or absent glucose and even whether white blood cells are present. Simply place one drop of CSF on each of the appropriate squares and read the results as if the CSF were urine. The use of urine reagent strips for diagnosing meningitis has been validated against standard techniques.

It is critical to establish an aetiology, particularly because of the risk of an epidemic of meningococcal meningitis. Gram-stain of CSF should be done if laboratory facilities are available. CSF should also be cultured.

If available, a latex agglutination test for meningococcal, pneumococcal and *Haemophilus* infections can be used for rapid detection of antigen in CSF. Note that false positives sometimes occur in patients with cerebral malaria. However, CSF protein and WCC are typically normal in cerebral malaria.

Other essential investigations

A blood film or rapid diagnostic test to exclude malaria would also be advisable.

Management of bacterial meningitis

If available, a third generation cephalosporin such as ceftriaxone or cefotaxime would be the antibiotic of choice. In many low-resource settings choice may be limited and chloramphenicol will often be the first-line recommendation.

For suspected pneumococcal meningitis, also give dexamethasone 0.15 mg/kg qds for 4 days. The first dose of dexamethasone should be given with or just before the first dose of antibiotics.

Bacterial meningitis in neonates

Give ampicillin and gentamicin or a third generation cephalosporin, such as ceftriaxone. If no alternative, chloramphenicol may be used but beware the risk of 'grey baby' syndrome particularly in pre-term or low birth-weight neonates. Be sure to adjust drug doses for weight and prematurity when prescribing in neonates.

Epidemic meningococcal meningitis
Oily chloramphenicol is the treatment of choice in epidemic meningococcal meningitis in Africa. A single dose of 100 mg/kg (maximum dose 3 g) given i.m. (half the dose into each buttock), is effective. The dose of oily chloramphenicol may be repeated after 24 hours if there is no clinical improvement. If after 48 hours there is still no improvement, treatment should be changed to either ceftriaxone or ampicillin. Oily chloramphenicol should not be used in pregnant women and children aged < 1 year for whom either ceftriaxone, ampicillin or standard chloramphenicol should be used instead.

Public health measures

The key question here is: Are we dealing with an epidemic of meningococcal disease? The scale of the public health response will be governed by incidence thresholds. Alert and epidemic thresholds have been defined by WHO for population sizes +/− 30 000. In this scenario, the population is < 30 000. Therefore, an alert threshold would be more than two cases/ week or an increase in number of cases compared to non-epidemic years. The 'alert' response is to inform the authorities, strengthen surveillance, investigate, confirm and treat cases and prepare for a possible epidemic. The 'epidemic' threshold for a population of < 30 000 would be either 'five cases/week' or 'doubling of the number of cases in a 3-week period'.

Chemoprophylaxis for close contacts of patients with meningococcal infections, although recommended in isolated cases or minor outbreaks, is not recommended by WHO in major epidemics.

Meningococcal vaccine
In the event of an epidemic, mass vaccination with an appropriate meningococcal polysaccharide vaccine should be initiated as soon as possible, with priority given to persons

aged 2–30 years. Mass vaccination will only influence the outcome of an epidemic if it is implemented within 5 weeks of the epidemic threshold being exceeded and an early intervention is unlikely to prevent more than half of expected cases. A new low-cost meningococcal A conjugate vaccine, which is safe and immunogenic in young children, is likely to replace the Group A polysaccharide vaccine in the future. Two doses as part of the EPI programme will offer protection for several years. A single dose targeting people aged 1–29 years is likely to be recommended in epidemic responses.

CASE STUDY 5

Fever in the highlands of Burundi, Africa

Situation – Highland Burundi; internally displaced person (IDP) camp. The nights are cold and conditions of hygiene are very poor. You have been asked to lead a health team to investigate an unusual febrile illness affecting people of all ages. Symptoms among the more severe cases have included rapid onset of high fever, severe headache and body pains, confusion, cough and breathlessness, meningism and a petechial rash. Initially this was thought to be an outbreak of meningococcal meningitis/septicaemia. However, CSF samples have been reported as normal by the laboratory which has facilities only for basic microscopy. Rapid diagnostic tests for malaria were negative. Blood films have also been reported as negative for malaria parasites. Furthermore, some patients with milder presentations have recovered without treatment after a few days only to have a further episode of fever a week or so later, and three patients with what appeared to be uncomplicated presentations suddenly deteriorated and died within a few hours of receiving treatment with an antibiotic.

What is the most likely cause of fever in these patients? How will you manage this situation?

Although there is a wide differential, louse-borne relapsing fever (LBRF) is the most likely diagnosis here. The clues are the epidemiological setting, clinical spectrum and progress and particularly the sudden deterioration of some cases following antibiotic treatment. Case fatality rates may approach 70 per cent in poorly managed epidemics.

LBRF is a multi-system disease that commonly presents with sudden onset chills, high fever, headache, myalgia, arthralgia, nausea, vomiting, dysphagia, dyspnoea and cough which may be productive of sputum containing *Borrelia*. Hepatomegaly, jaundice, splenomegaly (sometimes complicated by splenic rupture), albuminuria, petechiae, erythematous rash, epistaxis, conjunctival injection and haemorrhages, disseminated intravascular coagulation (DIC), confusion and meningism may also occur.

⚡ HAZARD

A potentially fatal Jarisch–Herxheimer reaction occurs in 80–90 per cent of treated LBRF cases, usually within a few hours of the first dose of antibiotic. It is characterized by severe rigors, restlessness and anxiety. An abrupt rise in temperature is associated with an initial tachycardia and increase in blood pressure followed by marked vasodilation and sweating, sometimes resulting in collapse and shock. Patients must be monitored closely in anticipation of this complication and may require intravenous fluids to maintain blood pressure. If available, meptazinol, an opioid antagonist, should be given to reduce the severity of the reaction. Steroids are of no benefit.

Complications include pneumonia, nephritis, arthritis, neuropathy, meningoencephalitis, meningitis, myocarditis, acute ophthalmitis, iritis and parotitis. Relapses occur after 5–9 days in two out of three cases and subsequently in a further one in four cases.

Diagnosis is made by identifying *Borrelia* (large spirochaetes) in Giemsa or Field stained blood films (often missed or a surprise finding in a patient with suspected malaria). The spirochaetes are also visible unstained using darkfield or phase-contrast microscopy.

Antibiotics

LBRF can be successfully treated with a single dose of antibiotic in about 95 per cent of cases. However, a 5–10 day course is usually prescribed to minimize the likelihood of relapses. Effective antibiotics include tetracycline, doxycycline, penicillin, erythromycin, chloramphenicol and ciprofloxacin. Ceftriaxone is recommended for patients with meningitis or encephalitis.

Louse-borne typhus (LBT)

LBT has many clinical features in common with LBRF. LBT is a multi-system, multi-organ disease characterized by microvascular thrombosis and perivascular infiltration. Therefore, clinical symptoms and signs may be very diverse. Case fatality rates tend to be low in children and increase with age if untreated reaching 50 per cent at 50 years. Severe cases may be complicated by DIC, myocarditis, respiratory problems associated with secondary infection and CNS involvement, including meningoencephalitis in 50 per cent of severe cases. CSF examination in such cases reveals raised protein and monocytes with normal glucose.

LBT also mimics meningococcal disease, including the development of petechial and haemorrhagic skin lesions and peripheral gangrene. Diagnosis is clinical and may be confirmed on serology. Dual infections of LBRF and LBT may occur. Preferred treatment is with doxycycline. Tetracycline, chloramphenicol, ciprofloxacin and rifampicin are also usually effective.

Control of louse-borne infections

This involves delousing clothing/bedding using insecticide powders, heat sterilization of clothing/bedding to kill eggs and personal delousing taking care not to crush the lice.

A word about viral haemorrhagic fevers

Depending on the epidemiological setting, viral haemorrhagic fevers (VHFs) may also need to be considered in the differential diagnosis for the above scenario and appropriate control measures implemented. In the case of yellow fever, this would include use of insecticide-treated bednets (ITNs) when nursing patients and mass immunization of the population at risk. In general, management of VHFs is supportive with administration of fluids (preferably ORS) and strict attention to minimizing risk of transmission via blood and body fluids. In addition, Lassa fever, Crimea-Congo haemorrhagic fever and Rift Valley fever may respond to early treatment with ribavirin.

Summary

Clinical work in low resource settings can be enormously challenging and hugely rewarding. Preparation is the key to success. MSF and other similar NGOs recommend specific training, for example the Diploma in Tropical Medicine and Hygiene programme at the Liverpool School of Tropical Medicine or the London School of Hygiene and Tropical Medicine. Time spent in the field working under the supervision and guidance of an experienced clinician will pay off when you face greater responsibility and isolation. Be prepared to listen, learn and take advice from your colleagues, your patients, members of their family and community. You won't have all the answers but you can go a long way towards finding effective solutions by asking the right questions, keeping an open mind and using your imagination and creativity. Try to maintain the highest professional standards possible, whatever the circumstances. Finally, remember that you will be a burden on others if you become ill or burn out, so take care of yourself.

FURTHER READING

Eddleston M, Davidson R, Brent A and Wilkinson R. *Oxford Handbook of Tropical Medicine* (3rd Edition). Oxford University Press, Oxford, 2005.

Gill G and Beeching N (eds). *Lecture Notes on Tropical Medicine* (6th Edition). Blackwell Scientific Publications, Oxford, 2009.

Websites

WHO

WHO Emergency Humanitarian Action website has excellent links including access to a huge range of electronic handbooks, manuals and emergency bibliography, many of which are also available on CD ROM. Of particular note is *Communicable Disease Control in Emergencies. A field manual.* Connolly MA (ed.) WHO, 2005.
www.who.int/hac/techguidance/en/

The WHO/PAHO *Health Library for Disasters* is also outstanding.
www.helid.desastres.net/

Integrated management of childhood illness (IMCI)
www.who.int/child_adolescent_health/documents/imci/en/index.html

Integrated management of adolescent and adult illness (IMAI)
www.who.int/3by5/publications/documents/imai/en/

Pocket book of hospital care for children
www.who.int/child_adolescent_health/documents/9241546700/en/index.html

MSF

Clinical Guidelines, Refugee Health, and other useful publications are available at: www.refbooks.msf.org/msf_docs/en/msfdocmenu_en.pdf

See also:

Clinical HIV/AIDS Care Guidelines for Resource-poor Settings (2nd Edition, 2006) Lynen L, MSF Belgium. Available at: telemedicine.itg.be/telemedicine/Uploads/MSF%20Guidelines%202006%2030 per cent20June%20MSF.pdf

7 Surgery in disasters

Jim Ryan

● Introduction

This chapter is concerned with the provision of surgical care in two of the most extreme environments known – on the battlefield and following a catastrophic natural disaster. At the time of writing there are over 50 wars taking place worldwide – the most recent additions to this woeful list are fresh conflicts in the north Caucasus, Southern Yemen and Somalia. Over 600 natural disasters are recorded annually affecting up to 150 million people. These events result in a variety of adverse health outcomes – surgeons have a key role.

In war and conflict there is usually a degree of early warning allowing planning and surgical assets are typically in place. The goals of the surgical response are well defined – provision of life- and limb-saving surgery for the wounded with the aim of conserving the fighting force. **Natural disasters typically occur without warning**, often involving the destruction or severe degradation of local medical resources. In this environment medical and surgical assets must be brought in by international humanitarian assistance teams to replace or augment local facilities and this takes time.

It is the provision of surgical care in the natural disaster environment that is the principal focus here. The goals of the surgical response in these settings are less clear compared to the battlefield and will be determined by many factors – these include timing of intervention, the nature of the disaster and the immediate needs as defined by an initial needs assessment. The common feature here is time lapse, often of days' duration or longer and this was well exemplified following the recent tsunami in Southeast Asia and earthquakes in Iran, Turkey, Pakistan and Haiti.

The objectives of an international surgical mission are myriad and diffuse and there is the risk of a long-term and open-ended commitment long after the immediate aftermath of the disaster event. An early and accurate *rapid needs assessment* is required before an effective response can be mounted.

HAZARD

Natural disaster hazards

Geophysical phenomena	**Weather phenomena**
Earthquakes	Tropical storms
Volcanoes	Floods
Tsunamis	Drought and famine
Land/mud slides	

● Needs assessment and planning the response

Conducting a rapid needs assessment requires early arrival at scene of a trained team with the correct mix of skills. **It is not for the amateur**. The United Nations has a specific agency for this purpose – the United Nations Disaster Assessment and Coordination Agency (UNDAC). Depending on the nature of the disaster an UNDAC team of two to six assessors is rapidly deployed to gather accurate intelligence and report on immediate needs and will submit an initial *rapid needs assessment* report.

The team's first task is to identify immediate threats to life (an impending epidemic for example) and assessment of the need to provide water, food, shelter and sanitation – the four immediate determinants of survival. The next priority is to identify emerging disease threats such as measles and diarrhoeal diseases. The team also considers local endemic threats such as malaria or viral haemorrhagic fevers. The surgical assessment, though urgent, is not the immediate concern of the UNDAC. However, where a surgical need is identified UNDAC will conduct an assessment and immediately report to international and non-government organizations (IOs and NGOs) specializing in surgical missions. These include the International Committee of the Red Cross (ICRC), Doctors Without Borders and Médicins Sans Frontières (MSF). A request for surgical input may come from other sources such as the health ministry of the affected country. Such a request was issued by the Sri Lanka health ministry to Leonard Cheshire International asking for an urgent assessment of surgical capability and capacity in the regions affected by the tsunami in December 1994. Another example was the request by the Philippines government to the US Air Force for assistance following the Mount Pinatabu earthquake in 1991.

There are other sources of information which inform UNDAC assessment teams. For example, there is a detailed and growing database for scores of natural and man-made disasters occurring over the last decade. This database is held by another UN agency – the UN Office for the Coordination of Humanitarian Affairs (OCHA). This information allows accurate prediction of injury for given disaster events.

● Use of OCHA database for predicting injury rates and patterns

Earthquakes
- High immediate mortality related to structural collapse, numbers of occupants, time of event and numbers trapped.

- Crush injury resulting in multiple fractures and renal failure.
- Injury to head, chest and abdomen rare in survivors.
- Timely extrication reduces mortality and morbidity.
- Fire risk to survivors.

Storms, floods and tsunamis

- Majority of deaths by drowning.
- Survivors present with inhalation injury and near-drowning.
- Complex limb fractures.
- Penetrating injury by glass, metal and wood debris in the water.

● Surgical needs assessment

Where an initial assessment by OCHA has identified surgical input a detailed surgical needs assessment **by surgeons** is vital in planning an appropriate response and to prevent the 'something must be done' approach which has blighted previous missions. The aim is to prevent inappropriate and indiscriminate despatching of surgical personnel and resources. The need for water, food, sanitation, housing and means to combat immediate health threats are constant for all disasters. The surgical response, however, will vary from mission to mission and its scope and extent and will be targeted to those in need and should await accurate intelligence.

The specific surgical needs assessment by an experienced surgical team is a two-part endeavour. An early rapid needs assessment by a small surgical team assesses the need for life- and limb-saving assistance and is carried out as soon as possible. Later, a second phase assessment is undertaken by specialist teams concerned with longer term needs exemplified by the need for plastic and reconstructive teams.

Figure 7.1 shows a multi-disciplinary, civil/military needs assessment team in Sri Lanka following the tsunami in 2004. There are broadly agreed guidelines for teams deploying to

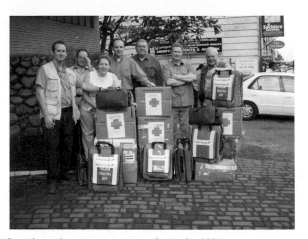

Fig. 7.1 Rapid needs assessment team Sri Lanka 2004.

conflict and disaster settings and these apply equally whether civilian or military. Team members must be field competent, self-sufficient in food, water, medical supplies, transport and communications. If necessary, a security element will be included. Collaboration with local authorities and with other deployed international teams is vital if duplication of effort and friction is to be avoided. Before beginning work senior team members must meet with senior health ministry officials and senior local surgical colleagues to receive an up-to-the-minute briefing as the situation on the ground changes by the hour in the immediate aftermath of a disaster. Key aims and objectives must be re-clarified and agreed by all parties.

In formulating the surgical priorities and activities, the surgical team leader must be aware of the wider picture in the disaster or conflict area and make decisions in the light of the overall health requirement as established by senior host and international aid agency officials. The leader must gain a clear appreciation of the nature and extent of the event, whether it is a natural disaster or a conflict setting. This must include estimates of the number killed, injured and those with urgent non-traumatic surgical need. In the case of an earthquake, for example, an estimate of the numbers trapped or missing is needed. There is also a need to understand the capability and capacity of the local response and of other deployed international teams. Based on this intelligence the team can develop its surgical strategy and recognize the need, if any, to request deployment of additional assets, both personnel and equipment.

● Executing the surgical response

THINKING POINT

In most situations, whether on the battlefield or following a natural disaster, immediate activities will be aimed towards care of the injured. Later the response may refocus to assist in the rehabilitation of host nation surgical services.

The skill mix of the team should be appropriate to the needs but typically the teams deployed initially consist of general and orthopaedic surgeons and support staff. In some settings and depending on accurate information, the team may be reinforced by obstetricians, paediatricians, nephrologists and critical care specialists. Decisions will also need to be made concerning additional training required to develop a self-sustaining team competent to work in an austere environment and on continuing medical and logistic support including re-supply.

Another area needing careful appraisal is work location – if local hospitals have been destroyed this will pose major logistic challenges. Tentage might be required – however, undamaged parts of affected hospitals may be used. Figure 7.2 shows a nephrology and critical care unit deployed in the basement of a wrecked hospital in Muzaffarabad, Pakistan following the earthquake in 2005. Further essential requirements include water and food security and a guaranteed 24-hour power supply.

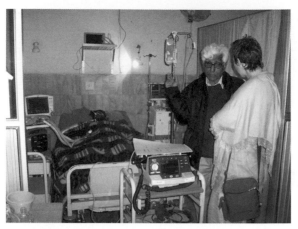

Fig. 7.2 ICU and renal dialysis setup in the basement of a destroyed hospital, Pakistan 2005.

Experienced medical experts (Hawley, 2002; Bricknell and MacCormack, 2005) have left detailed accounts of the act of medical intervention and are essential reading.

CLINICAL CONSIDERATIONS

Planning the surgical response – impacting factors

- Invitation and consent
- Achievable
- Security situation:
  - permissive
  - non-permissive
- Casualty estimates:
  - surgical illness
  - trauma – nature and numbers
- Host nation hospital infrastructure:
  - functional
  - compromised
  - destroyed
- State of host nation's surgical personnel:
  - numbers killed/injured

- uninjured and coping
- specific shortfalls – e.g. renal dialysis, plastic and reconstructive surgeons
- overwhelmed and exhausted

● Preparation and training

Working in a conflict or disaster environment is not for the enthusiastic amateur. The difficulty as we embark on the first decade of the 21st century is that there are few experts left in this field. The majority of first World surgeons have sub-specialized and few, if any, truly general surgeons remain. In the military this has resulted in what a distinguished former military professor of surgery calls 'surgeons hunting in teams'. Likewise on humanitarian deployments following natural disasters, team leaders now have to deploy larger teams to avoid gaps in competence. There is broad agreement that the absolute minimum a team should include would be a general surgeon, able to operate in the thorax as well as the abdomen and competent in basic vascular surgery techniques, and an orthopaedic surgeon, both with trauma experience.

L LEARNING POINTS

Deployed surgical team – basic competencies
- ATLS/BATLS qualified
- Triage competence
- Multi-system trauma resuscitation
- Surgical skill for the trauma patient – DSTS/DSTC qualified
- Critical care skills
- Command, organization and logistic basic skills
- Field craft

ATLS, Advanced Trauma Life Support; BATLS, Battlefield Advanced Trauma Life Support; DSTC, Definitive Surgical Trauma Course; DSTS, Definitive Surgical Trauma Skills.

Surgical team members are increasingly expected to have wider competencies. They may be expected to turn their hands to driving, watch-keeping, food preparation and even manual labour.

There are other important aspects to preparation before deployment. High motivation and physical and mental toughness are routine requirements for all teams, military and civilian. Increasingly, deploying agencies insist on pre-deployment assessment, training and testing.

● Clinical care in the early phase

Before the team has settled into its location, unpacked and set up to receive patients, an important decision should have been made concerning the scope and extent of the team's capability and how the team might most usefully contribute. A common error is to over-reach and embark on too ambitious an approach.

PEARL OF WISDOM

A wise decision is to limit care to what can be safely achieved – an experienced NGO surgeon tells prospective deploying surgeons, 'Stay in your lane' – this is excellent advice.

As a rule most teams should confine themselves, at least in the early stages, to trauma care and should avoid raising expectations or creating a culture of dependence. Later on, when the acute phase has passed it may be appropriate to widen the scope of care provided there is both the capability and capacity.

● Expected case mix

Surgical care in the immediate aftermath of most natural disasters involves treating large numbers of open, often complex fractures with associated soft tissue injuries. Because of numbers

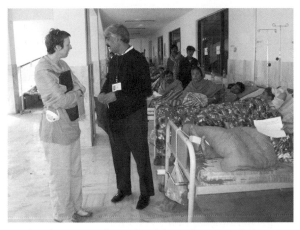

Fig. 7.3 Weighted traction achieved with bag of stones – Pakistan earthquake.

and relative shortages, a high degree of ingenuity is called for. Figure 7.3 shows an orthopaedic ward-round underway on a ward moved out of doors following the Pakistan earthquake. Note the femoral shaft fracture in the foreground treated by traction using a plastic bag full of stones.

Depending on the extent of delay in accessing care, many injuries will be neglected and, if open wounds are present, local and systemic infection will be evident further complicating care. Many limbs will be beyond salvage and an early decision to amputate is vital but demands experience and careful judgement. In others traumatic amputation will have occurred and the requirement here is careful management of the soft tissues and fashioning an appropriate stump.

CLINICAL CONSIDERATIONS

Wounds following injury on the battlefield or following natural disasters, an earthquake for example, have remarkable pathophysiological similarities – the time honoured military approach is appropriate for both – see page 168.

The guiding principles are those espoused by generations of military surgeons well versed in the management of multiple, complex penetrating and heavily contaminated wounds.

The military approach to contaminated wounds, irrespective of cause, is as follows:

- Preserve as much skin as possible – use a scrubbing brush to remove in-driven debris.
- In limb wounds perform fasciotomies along the entire limb length and not just confined to the extent of wounds. Consider counter incisions and counter fasciotomies on the side opposite the wound(s). When exploring wounds remember to open all deep fascial planes so as to comprehensively decompress the affected limb. This is the true definition of the widely misunderstood term – to debride. *Debridement* is a French word meaning to release or unbridle.
- Repair arteries essential for limb survival.
- Do not repair nerves at this stage but give consideration to marking injured nerve endings with a non-absorbable suture to aid late reconstruction.
- Dead and heavily contaminated soft tissue needs to be excised – again, experience and judgement are required.
- If bone fractures are present these require stabilization; however, internal devices should be avoided in the face of wound contamination – invariably present in these situations.
- Exposed joint cavities are particularly vulnerable to permanent deficit and must be meticulously washed out and covered by clean soft tissue.
- Finally, leave skin wounds and fasciotomies widely open. Dress wounds with layers of fluffed dry gauze, then overlay strips of gauze, then generous amounts of cotton wool followed by conforming stretch bandages.
- The limb, even when no fractures are present, should be stabilized on some form of splint for 3 to 4 days. After this time the wound should be re-inspected in the operating

room and, if clean, closed by suture, skin graft or a combination – this by tradition is called delayed primary suture (DPS).

⚡ **HAZARD**

In environments where entrapment and crush are prevalent – an earthquake is a common example – **crush syndrome and renal impairment must be expected** and poses particular challenges in austere settings. Inappropriate or uncontrolled release from entrapment may result in reperfusion leading to massive fluid sequestration, precipitating hypovolaemic shock. Myoglobinuria and hypovolaemia combine to cause acute renal failure requiring urgent renal dialysis.

Note, however, that even under the most difficult circumstances it is possible to create a critical care environment in the midst of disaster – go back to Figure 7.2. The ICU/dialysis team moved from Karachi on the day of the earthquake and set up in the basement of a partially destroyed teaching hospital. Within 24 hours a fully functioning ICU/renal dialysis unit was admitting patients.

● Clinical care – beyond the acute phase

Typically the role of a deployed surgical team will change when the acute phase has passed. Indeed many expatriate teams will return home. There is, however, much that can be achieved in the weeks and months that follow – but care and good planning is needed. The nature of the surgical requirement now changes – lengthy, costly and technically demanding reconstruction procedures by multi-disciplinary teams of orthopaedic and plastic surgeons are now needed – often for large numbers of people. In war this problem does not arise as wounded soldiers are evacuated back to the UK and are dealt with by the NHS. This is not possible following natural disasters and raises many difficulties.

Reconstructive work of this nature often hinges on specialized equipment such as operating microscopes and the availability of specialized physiotherapy and rehabilitation services – usually not available in disaster settings which typically occur in impoverished regions of the world.

Another trap also waits. The deployed team may at this time find themselves working alongside very experienced host nation surgeons who will assume the visiting team have appropriate competencies. **The rule is – state clearly your areas of competency.** 'Having a go' at procedures beyond the team's ability and competence will cause friction and bad feeling. Remarkably there are scores of examples where this has occurred.

A common task facing teams beyond the acute phase is to assist in the restoration of surgical and trauma services – this is a unique opportunity to make long-term contributions. Training and education are areas where effective help can be given at low cost. Joint case conferences and ward rounds are also valued by beleaguered local colleagues who value an opportunity to exchange ideas and demonstrate their own skills.

Summary

Joining a deployed surgical team, whether on a battlefield or following a natural disaster, affords unique opportunities, particularly relating to the difficulties faced by the host nation health system and by local colleagues. It is now commonplace for returning teams to act as advocates for the affected region – such advocacy must be driven by accurate data and not emotion. Governments, IOs and NGOs increasingly demand verifiable evidence before embarking on long-term rehabilitation missions.

REFERENCES

Bricknell MCM, MacCormack T. Military approach to medical planning in humanitarian operations. *British Medical Journal* 2005; **330**: 1437–9.

Hawley A. Health planning in action: Rwanda crisis. In: Hopperus–Buma APCC, Burris D, Hawley A, Ryan JM, Mahoney PF (eds). *Conflict and Catastrophe Medicine* (2nd Edition). Springer-Verlag, London, 2009, pp. 223–39.

8 Psychological aspects of conflict and catastrophe

Ian Palmer

● Introduction

This chapter will explore the psychological sequelae of exposure to conflict and catastrophe. It will draw attention to the importance of social interventions in the aftermath of disasters and touch upon the psychological constructs of the post-traumatic stress reaction.

Conflicts are man-made by design. Catastrophes may be man-made by accident or acts of nature (or God). Whatever the cause they disrupt the social fabric of families, communities, regions and even nations.

Akin to medical and surgical first aid, it is perhaps only natural to believe that mental health interventions should be deployed at an early stage of conflict and catastrophe if it is believed that all individuals exposed to toxic events will be psychologically damaged. Unfortunately there is little evidence that psychiatric interventions early in a catastrophe are of benefit to any other than those suffering from a formal psychiatric disorder at the time. Working with the self-selected populations that attend GP surgeries and hospitals is unlikely to teach doctors how catastrophe and conflict can bring out the best, and worst, in the human spirit. In conflicts and catastrophes survivors and helpers, individuals and groups can learn of what they are capable and can rise to moral and spiritual heights seldom seen in peace. Disasters affect groups and are therefore social and cultural experiences. Individuals behave differently in groups. Groups are stronger than the sum of their individuals. Therefore any mental health endeavour must be focused upon maintaining, supporting and encouraging social groups, helping them to pull together, to heal, to recover, rebuild and look to the future.

PEARL OF WISDOM

Conflicts and catastrophes are complex events that challenge societal, community and individual coping. Different disasters create different conditions for survivors and different specific realities which require addressing.

In communities affected by catastrophe it is of paramount importance not to pathologize normal human reactions to such events through the inappropriate use of western diagnostic criteria. Few doctors will be expert in recognizing normal as opposed to pathological human emotions unless they have worked outside their turf and comfort zone. It must be remembered that patients who attend psychiatric clinics are an even more rarefied patient group, and training with this population will benefit humanitarian aid, if those wishing to help focus their expertise and attention upon those individuals who have serious psychiatric disorders. It may be that general practitioners with an interest in psychological aspects of their patients will be of more use as they are more likely to be aware of the normal range of human experiences to loss and physical ailments. This whole issue is compounded when you are working in another's country. All professionals seeking to offer their services in support of conflict and catastrophe should work hard to avoid forming their own value judgements about normality and strive to understand the local population's and local experts' concepts of normality and patient management.

This said, there are a number of psychosocial phases to disasters (pre-impact, impact, recoil and post-impact).

● Psychosocial phases to disasters

Pre-impact phase

First, information may be available to communities prior to the disaster striking. Reactions to such information will relate to the type of the threat, previous experience of the threatened catastrophe, the sources of information and belief in the veracity of those sources as well as local rumour and gossip. In terms of mental health planning it will be important to recognize that those individuals with serious mental health problems in a community are more likely to require early intervention after the catastrophe strikes and perhaps even during the event(s). For individuals who have minor psychological or personality difficulties, early intervention is unlikely to be of benefit as the psychological sequelae in need of treatment following exposure to overwhelming events are likely to reveal themselves with the passage of time and/or degree of distress from the outset.

Impact and recoil phases

When disaster strikes individuals will initially react automatically to their situation and unlike the portrayal in Hollywood films, few panic unless individuals or groups believe escape is impossible. The danger of panic is its contagious nature; therefore anyone exhibiting it must be controlled rapidly for the benefit of the group. About one in ten may be ineffective but about one in four will remain effective and emotionally well-controlled and may be of inestimable value at the time. Most individuals will exhibit a wide range of psychological reactions; however, with appropriate guidance and direction from members within the community or external support, may be galvanized into productive action. When a disaster strikes there is an 'illusion of centrality' – individuals believe that they are at the centre of the disaster. Emotions run strong and range from disbelief and numbness to confusion and fear of death. Survival behaviours require cooperation, courage, heroism and altruism seldom seen in times of peace.

Post-impact phase

The challenge in all humanitarian aid is how to get there quickly and save lives while respecting local customs and recognizing positive local structures and individuals to ensure intervention does not create dependency. Initially there will be a honeymoon period as a life resembling normality is attempted. This may be replaced by covert or overt feelings of resentment and hostility at what has happened and towards those who are offering help or those who are better off, particularly if felt to be arrogant or imperialistic in their ways. **Anger should be understood and channelled into useful action, unlike dependency and despondency**.

Even with the best will, promises made at the outset may not be followed through and those in receipt of aid will experience feelings of abandonment, disillusionment, disappointment and resentment that the world has forgotten them. By this time, communities will realize that it is up to them to reconstruct with whatever help is remaining. Sadly, criminality and corruption are frequent, sometimes endemic and only add to their communities' problems. Accommodation to a disaster believed to be man-made is usually more problematic for individuals and groups than if the disaster was an act of nature. The prospect of someone being responsible allows the projection of distress, anger and pain on to a clearly-defined individual or group akin to scapegoating. The identification of a responsible other also offers the prospect of revenge, retribution and justice for such loss. Sadly, however, a continued focus on blame and retribution over forgiveness, reconciliation and reconstruction can only delay healing in both individuals and groups. Vested political and media interests have both malign and positive impact in survivor communities. **Time is a potent healer particularly when allied with constructive occupation and investment**.

At an individual level there are consistent issues of guilt and shame. For some the elation of survival is replaced by guilt. Frequently there are ruminations about acts of omission or commission. Bereavements and the spiritual accompaniments of death will be important challenges for both individuals and communities. It is therefore important to know at which phase of the disaster you are offering your services. The most appealing time is likely to be in the acute phase, however, the most benefit may occur later. This also gives a message that these individuals are not forgotten by the outside world.

Since World War I, there has been an inexorable rise in civilian casualties. Some organizations now target civilians. War means bereavement for combatants, families and communities. War involves atrocity. War requires healing, reconciliation, reintegration, reconstruction and rebuilding of social structures. The external threat of conflict may lead to increased social cohesion in different parts of the community or nation. As conflicts grow their impact on the fabric of society grows. Although the psychological cost will be felt by few, it will be over-reported and lead to anxieties in others, particularly those predisposed to such concerns. At an individual level it is important to remember that post-traumatic stress disorder is not the most common post-traumatic mental disorder encountered in survivors of catastrophes. The most common psychological outcome is no mental health disorder.

HAZARD

Mental health professionals consistently underestimate emotional resilience in the face of great adversity. While everyone is changed by traumatic experiences, recovery is the norm. Be clear why you are involved in this work and how not to (re-)traumatize those you seek to help by application of inappropriate psychological models of care and intervention.

● Interventions

In both conflict and catastrophe there is little point in attempting any mental health interventions until individuals and communities are safe and feel safe. Thus social interventions are the most important aimed at providing safety, clean water, shelter, normality and routine. Social structures are important in good mental and social health – they support individuals during crisis and afterwards, thus it is important to strive to reconstitute disrupted family, kinship and cultural groups as soon as possible. Individuals and communities will have lost many material, emotional and spiritual possessions. Focus on resilience and strengths are vital for healing individuals and groups. Losses must be acknowledged and, when appropriate, time set aside to mourn them. Solutions not problems are the focus.

CLINICAL CONSIDERATIONS

During the acute phase of the disaster, the emphasis should be on social interventions. Following conflict and catastrophe the most important psychological interventions are social – safety, shelter, food and water, occupation, routine and healing.

Effective mental health interventions require understanding, recognition and respect for local culture, traditions and belief systems. As a guest it is important to work with existing community social and psychiatric providers to provide sensitive, empowering and achievable aid. Western mental health specialists may be best employed back at base locations allowing those who understand local requirements and facilities go forward into the disaster area to provide culturally appropriate support and intervention. In many parts of the world there are few mental health workers and even fewer psychiatrists and thus it may be of benefit to train local population health workers to manage and triage any mental health requirements.

Disasters are experienced at an individual, community, national and international level. Disasters affect groups. Few doctors have experience of working with groups. Individuals behave differently in groups. Groups have membership rules and will endeavour to heal themselves. Groups will tend to avoid pathologizing normal (human) cognitive, emotional and behavioural reactions in their members.

While everyone is changed to varying degrees by their experiences of conflict or catastrophe only a few are damaged. Although inevitable and irrevocable, change following adversity need not be negative; indeed mental health professionals consistently underestimate individual and group emotional resilience in the face of great adversity.

● Post-traumatic symptom aetiology

Mental disorders, even serious and enduring mental illnesses, are multi-factorial in aetiology. They are the product of an interaction between the individual or group, life events (stressors), the environment and the culture in which this individual lives. Individuals have genetic, social and psychological predispositions to mental ill-health. Those from deprived backgrounds are disproportionately represented in mental health services. Individuals who have a history of psychiatric disorder, personality problems and concurrent difficulties are more likely to develop mental disorders. However, at times of great adversity, some will overcome their disadvantages and function well.

Survivor communities focus on the future and current survival needs more than contemplating past events. PTSD symptoms decline with time and only a minority will develop post-traumatic mental disorder. As the post-trauma environment shapes the trajectory of post-traumatic symptoms, post-disaster interventions should focus on communal psychosocial needs, improving social networks, regenerating interpersonal bonds, community coherence, gainful employment and an effective system of justice where possible. There is unlikely to be a need for individual-centred psychological interventions. **Psychiatric focus should concentrate on those with current mental disorders and the long-term detection of those with continuing difficulties**.

The individual

The individual with all of their variability, experiences, vulnerabilities and strengths will interact uniquely with toxic or traumatic events. The interaction is complex and mediated through meaning which is dependent on current mental state, past experiences, current situation, individuals and cultural beliefs and practices as well as education. Meaning is a dynamic process leading to different appraisals at different stages, e.g. survivors or victims.

Toxic events (stressors)

Stressors are also uniquely variable. Generally, the more traumatic the event the more likely it is to lead to psychological distress but seldom does the intensity or type of stressor predict the likelihood of an individual developing a post-traumatic mental disorders such as PTSD.

Thus both individuals and stressors are infinitely variable and meaning mediates the interaction. Toxic events are usually unexpected, even when 'expected', e.g. hurricanes. They are **loss** events, e.g. loss of loved ones, possessions, communities, predictability and routine. They may be repetitive and hold individuals close to the belief that they are just about to die (the duration of this experience is particularly 'traumatogenic'). Individuals may undergo grotesque sensory experiences involving disgust and revulsion, particularly olfactory assault, which remain powerful triggers to later re-experiencing phenomena perhaps because it is memorized in the palaeoencephalon. Events may be experienced as an individual or as a group. Military groups serve to protect their members from succumbing to overwhelming experiences at the time through their structure and over-learnt behaviours (drills). Toxic stressors may be man-made or natural. Man-made disasters cause more problems than natural ones.

The post-trauma environment

This shapes the trajectory of post-traumatic symptoms. The environment is thus an important variable during and after exposure. In general, individuals who experience adversity in a group may benefit from the shared group 'experience' at the time and afterwards particularly when the group is strong and mutually supportive. 'Adversity' groups (those brought together by chance or fate) are generally less helpful over time as they are less homogenous and there has been no investment in group membership before the toxic event. 'Given' groups offer a better prospect for support and healing but even they can have difficulties if the event disrupts the group dynamic, e.g. leaders who let the group or community down in crisis. This said, commeth the day, commeth the (wo)man and natural leaders may emerge who help move the community forward. Depending on the disaster, communities may experience isolation and ostracism from neighbours within their nation, as in Chernobyl and Nagasaki for example.

The environment plays a significant role in the development of post-trauma mental ill-health. At the individual level, the environment contains social contacts (family, friends, workmates) who play a key role in recovery. This can be a complicated affair as the narrative presented by the survivor is likely to be different to different audiences – household pets probably hear a lot more than doting grandparents.

Having come through unpleasant experiences few will wish to 'traumatize' loved ones by telling the whole truth. Some audiences want to hear different stories, for example youths frequently ask soldiers what it's like to kill someone. Journalists will seek out the unusual for a 'scoop' and 'good copy'. We in the West believe that talking helps but only talking when the individual or group is ready – this can take months or even years. Sometimes talking, even with those with whom the stressor was shared, may not be enough and professional help should be sought. And we should not forget; some narratives are false.

PEARL OF WISDOM

It is important not to pathologize normal human emotional reactions to unpleasant events.

Grief and bereavement are culturally-shaped rituals and processes and useful paradigms for the management of post-trauma mental distress and disorder which, like grief, can be simple or complicated and generally settle within a finite period of time for most people. Grief 'work' is the social and cultural process of coming to terms with and accommodating to loss in the form of death. In most circles, other than journalism, the grieving process is recognized as an intensely personal experience for families and friends. External intrusion can interfere with the process. Exposure to traumatic events also leads to loss: loss of things we normally take for granted, for example existential omnipotence, faith in the predictability of life, faith itself and the like. Post-trauma 'work' may thus be thought of as accommodating (psychologically, socially and culturally) to these changes. Some bereaved require professional advice and support; so it is with post-trauma stress reactions.

As with bereavement, the post-traumatic healing can be disturbed by external intrusion. Unlike most deaths, traumatic events are newsworthy and court intrusion to feed the voracity of the 24-hour networks. Survivors will be sought for their narrative. Some will talk, others won't. The events, however, and thus the individual's experience, will become public property, the centre of conjecture, debate and comment by 'experts' who weren't there. Seldom is this therapeutic for the individual, family or community. Media interest is, however, transient as they are not there for the long haul – it isn't 'good copy'.

Culture

Thus culture is the fourth variable involved in the development of mental disorders. In Western medicine there is a focus on problems and individuals' weaknesses and vulnerabilities, rather than their strengths and resilience. Media commentators would have us believe that almost anyone exposed to almost any unpleasant experience is psychologically damaged and in need of specialist help. This is untrue. The majority of individuals exposed to the same unpleasant events will cope adequately and may perhaps even benefit from experience.

● Post-traumatic stress symptoms

In the West there is extant an 'urban myth' that PTSD is the only, or the most common psychological reaction following exposure to extreme stressors; it isn't. Anxiety, depression and substance misuse are much more common.

The three pillars of the post-trauma response are re-experiencing, arousal and avoidance. The symptoms are not uncommon and are generally short-lived (usually settling within 12 weeks). For some individuals, however, they may be severe and associated with other psychiatric symptoms. It is difficult to tell when a reaction becomes a disorder after trauma and the labels acute stress disorder and PTSD remain controversial and the focus of continuing debate.

A moment's introspection will reveal that the phenomena of re-experiencing, arousal and avoidance are part of a common human experience reflected in everyday language. For example, we all know what is meant when someone says they have 'something on their mind', they feel 'wound up' or 'on edge' or are trying 'to put things to the back of their mind'. We have all had these experiences and perhaps it is unsurprising that the worse the stressor, the more we have to ruminate on a problem in order to make sense of what has been happening to us. The worse the stressor, the more likely we are to try to put things out of our mind and avoid talking about them as it distresses us.

We are also more likely to avoid situations, people and places that are likely to trigger our distress. The more distressed we become, the worse we sleep, the more irritable and edgy we feel and the more likely we are to seek solace in alcohol or other substances to soothe our arousal.

Individuals (and groups) cope with experiences using processes that have worked for them before. Unsurprisingly, the worse the event the greater these experiences are likely to be. The only clear evidence for treating problematic post-traumatic stress reactions or disorder is for exposure therapies. Once the unpleasant events are revisited their power is lessened and arousal diminishes. Sometimes it takes time to find the right person to trust enough to share the experience with. It is a serious mistake to attempt to try to **make** an individual talk about their experiences – as with grief, there is a time to talk. At the outset of the PTSD debate, it was felt that early inter-vention with psychological debriefing was useful. This was erroneously based on misinterpreted military experiences of the management of acute breakdown in combat. The military post-operational debriefing process and observation from police work demonstrates that everyone experiences unpleasant events differently. The initial recommendation was to get everyone who experienced unpleasant events together and talk about it in a group so that they would be able to process the events better, which would prevent the development of PTSD. Unfortunately this process underestimated or ignored the ingrained coping mechanisms of individuals and only served to over-arouse those involved so that it was more difficult to process the information from a heightened emotional state created by the debriefing process itself, generally carried out by an outsider who was not there.

Most post-traumatic stress reactions settle within three months so a 'wait and see' policy isn't a bad idea. However, those deeply disturbed from the outset and those who do not improve or who get worse after about three months may benefit from pro-fessional help. Some individuals may require tranquillizing medication akin to pain relief for a broken bone. Individuals may apply their own emotional pain relief by way of alcohol or drugs, which may add to their problems if misuse continues over time. It is most important not to confuse late psycho-therapeutic interventions with those required soon after a traumatic event. In time of crisis public, rather than individual, mental health is important. Safety, succour and social support are the lynch-pins of this. Indeed, **'there are hardly any relevant public health promotional measures which require expertise in client-centred psychological help'**.

● Get involved

For those contemplating going to help out during or after a conflict or catastrophe, it is important to remember that your role is to support and, where possible, create community pro-cesses that allow and empower individuals and groups to achieve control and autonomy over their situation. You do not need to be trained in psychology and psychiatry to do this and, unless you have other skills to offer, you may be a burden – in a crisis it's all hands to the pumps and if you want to do psychiatry, earn credibility by joining in the community effort. Physical safety and shelter are the most important first steps.

Psychological first aid involves 'being there' and 'bearing witness' to human suffering with compassion, simple human warmth and kindness. Identifying and working alongside those who support the social, cultural and spiritual well-being of the community is fundamental to your credibility and acceptance from the outset. Tracing and reuniting orphans, families and friends is a crucial part of recovery. Work is good for you and the communities you will serve. It is important to identify purposeful, concrete and shared work to be undertaken communally. Work empowers individuals and mitigates any potential for dependency on aid.

Whatever your level of skill you will always have something to learn from people who live in these communities and it is important to work with professional colleagues, local health workers and healers and non-medical carers to provide what **they** think is most important for their communities. You are not there for you; you're there for them. It is important to encourage pride, self-sufficiency and avoid dependency at every step.

CASE STUDY

Rwanda vignettes – following the Genocide

- In one location each of the village elders had lost at least four family members to the killing. Their bodies were coming to the surface of the shallow graves in which they were hastily interred by local families and becoming a health hazard as children were playing with body parts. As part of the UN we sought a way of helping this process. At every turn our suggestions were agreed and it took a long time to find out what was really required. We tried to be sensitive to spiritual/ religious desires only to find out that it didn't matter what we did as there could be no peace for the murdered souls till the Diaspora returned. What they wanted us to do was to try to stop massive NGO food trucks careering through their village every day of the week – they wanted Sunday kept free of this traffic so they could meet and grieve in peace and not risk injury from trucks badly driven at high speed through their village.

- I met with women survivors in Kigali with Bishop Jonathan to explore the possibility of bringing women together therapeutically. No women thought this a good idea. All had had too much loss and grief to deal with and could not bear to add to this by listening to other women's stories. About 10 years later such groups were in existence.

- In one village where a particularly dreadful massacre had occurred, the establishment of a school for the children was a most powerful therapeutic intervention. Many children had survived under the dead bodies of their parents and were starting the process of healing through art. The school also gave purpose to the grown-ups working there, many of whom were having more difficulty than the children. Establishment of work, routine and community are powerful therapeutic tools in recovery.

- **Aid work is not easy.** Accommodating to differing values and mores can be challenging. Working to 'head office' directions can cause friction especially when plans require frequent revision in response to changing local situations. Criminality, organized crime and corruption are endemic in some parts of the globe and potentially very dangerous for not only you but also local populations. Sometimes the most important psychological intervention will be to record atrocities and corruption and inform the appropriate national or international bodies.
- **It is important to get as much information as possible prior to deploying abroad.** Information gleaned from the media will be biased so, if at all possible, it is important to speak to people who have recently been to the theatre of operations.
- **You will achieve more as part of a team**, especially if you have a chance to train with them prior to deployment. Any effort spent in building team cohesion is never wasted – it will act as a social and psychological resource for team members and will enhance your capabilities on the ground. Once deployed, everyone should be made aware of their role in the big picture. Regular rest periods must be taken and total time on unpleasant tasks rigidly controlled. Disasters are very confusing and plans seldom last very

long so flexibility is vital. It is important that those who have specific training and skills should be able to use these to the best benefit of the host nation.

Emotionally it is important at the end of each day to have an opportunity (whether taken or not) to talk about what's happened during the day. Individuals' personal coping styles must be respected and groups should set time aside to enjoy themselves and rest properly. This will feel (and probably sounds) a bit odd but, without attention to management of staff well-being, their interventions may become less effective and individuals run the risk of 'burn out'. Socializing and sharing are important for group dynamics, health and cohesion. While many individuals use alcohol and drugs recreationally without detriment there is always the risk of their use masking psychological problems, or creating inter-personal problems (arguments, violence, sex) which can alter the group dynamic and interfere with effectiveness and compromise the achievement of the mission. Sexual relationships are common, can become very intense and have after-effects for partners on return but no one has yet figured out a way to prevent this happening.

Identification of those having trouble can be as simple as noticing a change in personality or character. Such changes may signify problems such as substance misuse, burn-out, depression, etc. Well-run teams should respect each other and that bringing attention to such change is a function of 'mateship' and not a personal attack. **This said, it is easy neither to impart nor receive such information**. Disturbance in bodily drives (sleeping, eating, libido); irritability; inability to settle; anxiety; indecisiveness are signs others will notice – the outward manifestation of more intra-psychic distress known only to the individual. Some individuals are more psychologically-minded than others but it is important for all who undertake aid work to know where they can seek help on return – any reputable NGO will have access to such help for their returning aid-workers. It is also important to remember to seek help any time during or after return – it works.

Undertaking aid work will change you; hopefully for the better. Those left behind will change in your absence. Disaster work will be challenging, at times deeply rewarding, at other times deeply distressing but most individuals cope well.

THINKING POINTS

- When does a normal human reaction become a mental disorder?
- How would you prepare for work in Humanitarian Aid?
- Under what circumstances would you consider going with an NGO?
- What narrative would you construct on your return and for whom?

Summary

- Hardly any relevant public health promotional measures require expertise in client-centred psychological help.
- Mental health professionals should help local mental health colleagues aid those currently psychiatrically unwell within the community and, in the medium to long term, assist in detection of and help for those with continuing difficulties consequent upon their exposures.
- Disasters are experienced at an individual, community, national and international level. Psychological phases of natural disasters include pre-impact; impact; recoil, recovery, reconstruction and rebuilding.

- Social rather than psychiatric measures are more important in the reconstitution of societies following catastrophe and include help to establish an effective system of justice.
- Exposure to toxic events and psychological sequelae are not a direct cause and effect. They are a product of an interaction between the infinite variables of: the individual, the stressors, the environment (at the time and afterwards) and culture from which the survivors come and to which they return.
- Any mental health intervention requires understanding, recognition and due cognisance of local culture, traditions and belief systems, and to be effective needs to build upon, and work with, existing community support mechanisms that remain, however tenuous they may be.
- Conflicts and catastrophes strike groups. Few doctors have experience of working with groups or understanding of how differently individuals behave in groups, how groups endeavour to heal themselves and how important it is for group membership to avoid pathologizing normal human cognitive, emotional and behavioural reactions.
- It must be remembered from the outset that, while everyone is changed by their experiences to a greater or lesser extent, recovery from major traumatic events is the norm and mental health professionals consistently underestimate emotional resilience in the face of great adversity. Such exposure may lead to positive change in individuals and communities.

FURTHER READING

Thematic papers. Natural disasters and their aftermath. *International Psychiatry* 2006; **3** (3).

Alexander DA. Early mental health intervention after disasters. *Advances in Psychiatric Treatment* 2005; **11**: 12–18.

Palmer I. Psychosocial costs of war in Rwanda. *Advances in Psychiatric Treatment* 2002; **8**: 17–25.

Van Ommeren M, Saxena S and Saraceno B. Aid after disasters. *BMJ* 2005; **330** (7501): 1160–1.

Hodgkinson PE and Stewart M. *Coping with Catastrophe: a handbook of post-disaster pyschological aftercare* (2nd Edition). Brunner-Routledge, London, 1998.

Committee on Treatment of Posttraumatic Stress Disorder. Institute of Medicine of the National Academies. *Treatment of Post Traumatic Stress Disorder: an assessment of the evidence*. The National Academes Press, Washington DC, 2007. Available at: www.nap.edu/catalog.php?record_id=11955 (Accessed: 19 July 2008).

Department of Health. *International Humanitarian and Health Work: toolkit to support good practice*. Department of Health, London, 2003. Available at: www.dh.gov.uk/prod_consum_dh/groups/dh_digitalassets/@dh/@en/documents/digitalasset/dh_4074576.pdf (Accessed: 19 July 2008).

9 Marginalized groups in disasters

Maria Kett

● Introduction

This chapter will give the reader an overview of aspects to take into consideration when thinking about planning, intervening and assisting with recovery from disasters and where to find more in-depth advice and guidelines. Although these groups are often discussed as 'vulnerable groups', in many ways this is a misleading title – in the event of a disaster, all of us are vulnerable to a greater or lesser degree. Some, however, are more marginalized and excluded than others. It is these people, who have the least capacity and resources to protect and sustain themselves, that this chapter will focus on.

● Who, What, When, Where and Why?

Who?

As noted above, everyone can be considered at risk in a disaster or emergency, but some groups are more likely to be at risk. These include:

- women
- children
- older adults
- people with disabilities

- minority groups (e.g. ethnic, cultural, linguistic, religious groups; pastoralists)
- refugees and internally displaced people (IDPs)
- people living with HIV/AIDS

It is these groups that the second half of this chapter will focus on.

What and why?

Of what and why are these groups at more specific risk?

- invisibility (including lack of political representation or power)
- discrimination, stigma and prejudice (by communities and by those providing relief programmes)
- lack of awareness (by agencies and organizations)
- lack of data or information (including definitions and categorization)
- assumptions (for example, that there is already someone to look after them; or that targeted assistance is expensive)
- lack of participation (often linked to misconceptions about abilities)
- lack of priority (for example, for child protection programmes)
- poverty (often linked to many of the above problems and meaning less likelihood of other protective mechanisms such as insurance being available)
- increased risk of violence (especially toward women and children)
- media representation (for example, of risks associated with dealing with people living with HIV).

When and where?

Because of the marginalization and disenfranchisement they experience, many members of these groups are less likely to be engaged in income-generating activities, education, or to be linked into wider community support structures, or be linked to social protection schemes. Therefore traditional support

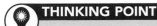

THINKING POINT

As examples from recent events, such as the Indian Ocean tsunami in 2004, and the Haiti and Chile earthquakes in 2010 have demonstrated, disasters can and do affect anyone; however, these events have also shown that the more a group is marginalized, the more vulnerable to the effects of disasters they are.

mechanisms, such as material resources, family and friends may not be available but also other protective structures such as insurance may be lacking. In the event of a disaster, already vulnerable people are then among the worst affected. It is also vital to remember that none of these are homogenous groups and people can be even further excluded and marginalized, for example on the basis of gender, religion or ethnicity.

How?

So what can be done by agencies and organizations working in the area of Disaster Medicine to better ensure that marginalized groups are included in responses? There cannot be a 'one size fits all approach'; however, it should be remembered that overall, each person has the same basic needs (water, food, shelter, etc.), but what differs are the approaches used to provide these and some modifications or extra services and support may be needed.

It is vital to remember that any humanitarian intervention is bound by international humanitarian law and there are a number of international laws and conventions in place to ensure the protection of marginalized groups. This is the cornerstone of the work of the International Disaster Response Laws, Rules and Principles (IDRL) programme, which seeks to reduce vulnerability and marginalization through awareness and strengthening and implementing rule of law for disaster responses. It ensures legal preparedness for disasters through national disaster preparedness, response and recovery frameworks (see Table 9.1 and www.ifrc.org/what/disasters/idrl/).

Table 9.1 Key legal frameworks for protection

International Convention on the Elimination of All Forms of Racial Discrimination (1965)

International Covenant on Economic, Social and Cultural Rights (1966)

International Covenant on Civil and Political Rights (1966)

Refugee Convention (1951 and 1967 Protocol)

Convention on the Elimination of All Forms of Discrimination against Women (1979)

Convention on the Rights of the Child (1989)

Convention on the Rights of Persons with Disabilities (2008)

The following are not legally binding but have had significant impact on protection issues internationally:

Universal Declaration of Human Rights (1948)

Declaration on the Elimination of Violence Against Women (1993)

Declaration on the Rights of Indigenous Peoples (2007)

Guiding Principles on Internal Displacement (1998)

PEARL OF WISDOM

In today's world, when a disaster strikes, responses are global. It is rare that any sovereign state refuses offers of international assistance.

● Whose responsibility?

The UN has played a vital role in taking the lead in responses to disasters, from its inception following World War II to its current humanitarian reform programme. The agency charged with coordinating UN responses to disasters and emergencies across the world is the Office for the Coordination of Humanitarian Affairs (OCHA). OCHA is headed by the Emergency Relief Coordinator (ERC). The ERC is also chair of the Inter-Agency Standing Committee (IASC), which was established in 1992 in response to a UN Resolution to strengthen humanitarian assistance. The IASC is made up of UN organizations, the International Committee of the Red Cross and Red Crescent (ICRC); the International Federation of Red Cross and Red Crescent Societies (IFRC) as well as a number of other non-UN humanitarian partners.

The Cluster System

In order to facilitate the process of strengthening humanitarian assistance, a new system, known as the 'Cluster System', has been introduced in a number of humanitarian situations (both immediate and ongoing) around the world. The overall aim of the cluster system is to eliminate the deficiencies that were found in earlier humanitarian responses. Each sector – or 'cluster' – is led by a UN body which takes overall responsibility for preparedness, technical capacity coordination and final responsibility for provision and accountability of the sector (see Table 9.2). The Global Clusters are led by the ERC, who designates a Humanitarian Coordinator (HC) for each specific disaster or emergency response in agreement with the IASC.

The overall aim of these reforms is to make humanitarian responses more effective, more coordinated and above all, more accountable; however, this last point also necessitates that the lead agency is 'provider of last resort' – that is, if no one else can provide the service, the Global Cluster Lead must. For example, the Global Health Cluster consists of over 30 international humanitarian health organizations, led by the WHO. The aims of the Cluster System are in line with the general aims of humanitarian reform, as well as having a focus on strengthening national capacity of preparedness, response and resilience to disasters. It is the issue of provision and accountability, however, that has led the IFRC, to act as convenor only, as they argue that the chain of accountability contravenes their seven key principles, particularly those of independence and neutrality. At country level, MSF have voiced similar concerns.

The chart in Table 9.2 describes the 11 Clusters and the Global Cluster Leads (see also www.humanitarianreform.org/humanitarianreform/Default.aspx?tabid=70).

Table 9.2 Global Cluster Leads

Sector or area of activity	Global Cluster Lead
Agriculture	FAO
Camp coordination/management: IDPs (from conflict)	UNHCR
Disaster situations	IOM
Early recovery	UNDP
Education	UNICEF
	Save The Children – UK
Emergency shelter: IDPs (from conflict)	UNHCR
Disaster situations	IFRC (Convener)
Emergency telecommunications	OCHA/UNICEF/WFP
Health	WHO
Logistics	WFP
Nutrition	UNICEF
Protection: IDPs (from conflict)	UNHCR
Disasters/civilians affected by conflict (other than IDPs)	UNHCR/OHCHR/UNICEF

FAO, Food and Agricultural Organization; IDPs, internally displaced persons; IFRC, International Federation of Red Cross and Red Crescent; IOM, International Organization for Migration; OCHA, Office for the Coordination of Humanitarian Affairs; OHCHR, Office of the High Commissioner for Human Rights; UNDP, United Nations Development Program; UNHCR, United Nations High Commissioner for Refugees; UNICEF, United Nations International Children's Emergency Fund; WFP, World Food Program; WHO, World Health Organization.

In addition, the UN has identified four issues that cut across all of the 11 Global Clusters. These are age, gender and HIV. This list is not exhaustive but represents a commitment to integrate often-excluded and vulnerable groups.

It is also important to note and relevant to the discussion here, that the global situation is not necessarily replicated at country level. For example, while the United Nations High Commissioner for Refugees (UNHCR) is the lead of the global Protection Cluster, at country level in disaster situations or in complex emergencies without significant displacement, one of the three core protection-mandated agencies (UNHCR, United Nations International Children's Emergency Fund [UNICEF] or the Office of the High Commissioner for Human Rights

[OHCHR]) will liaise with the designated HC and decide who will be the lead organization.

● General guidelines

It should also be noted that as well as the overall humanitarian reforms, there have been a number of initiatives to improve the effective planning and delivery of humanitarian aid, following a number of incidences when aid delivery did not have the intended consequences. These are well-publicized and include the situation in the camps in Goma (in former Zaire) following the Rwandan Genocide in 1994, where many agencies realized that the food and other aid they were providing was being diverted to the *genocidaires* and not to the people most in need (Goodhand, 2006). This led to attempts to provide guidelines not only on the practical delivery of humanitarian aid, but also on the ethics and principles. One of the most well known of these is the Sphere Project.

Sphere Project: Humanitarian Charter and minimum standards in disaster response

The Sphere Project (www.sphereproject.org/) is a voluntary network of organizations, including the ICRC, UN organizations, donors, government representatives, representatives from affected populations and other NGOs who collaborate to undertake a commitment to quality and accountability and produce a handbook that can be used in the field to ensure these are carried out to the best minimum standards.

L **LEARNING POINT**

The Sphere Standards are based on two fundamental principles: the necessity to take all possible measures to alleviate suffering in situations of disasters and conflict; and that all those affected by disasters have a right to life with dignity and a right to assistance.

These principles described above have been derived from:

- International Humanitarian, Human Rights and Refugee law
- The Code of Conduct: Principles of Conduct for the International Red Cross and Red Crescent Movement and NGOs in Disaster Response Programmes.

In addition to the Sphere Project, the IASC also produces a number of other field guides and reports based on broad consensus within the humanitarian community and endorsed by the IASC Working Group or IASC Principals, which are used by humanitarian actors in the field or in policy work. A full list of all products is available from the IASC website and can be downloaded free of charge: (www.humanitarianinfo.org/iasc/content/products/default.asp).

These include:

- IASC Guidelines on Mental Health and Psychosocial Support in Emergency Settings
- Women, Girls, Boys and Men. Different Needs – Equal Opportunities: IASC Gender Handbook for Humanitarian Action
- IASC Operational Guidelines and Field Manual on Human Rights Protection in Situations of Natural Disaster
- IASC Operational Guidelines on Human Rights and Natural Disasters
- IASC Guidelines on Gender-Based Violence Interventions.

Women and children

It is important to examine both men's roles and the relations between men and women, in different situations. Nor will merely undertaking acts such as ensuring that areas like paths and latrines in camps are well lit (although these measures are necessary) ensure gender equity or empowerment as this does not address some of the fundamental issues of power and exclusion that may be present.

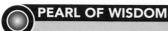

PEARL OF WISDOM

It is important to note that any discussion around gender issues should not solely focus on women.

The number of issues confronting children – including adolescents and youths – in disasters is vast and ranges from forced conscription and child labour through to education and employment. **It is therefore important to consider issues of marginalization and exclusion within a family and a community context.**

It is now well-recognized that women and children do have specific capabilities and requirements in situations of emergency and disaster. In addition to the general guidelines listed above, there are a number of resources that specifically focus on women and children. There are a number of organizations mandated to advance the position of women: the United Nations Development Fund for Women (UNIFEM), the UN body charged with responsibility for gender issues (www.unifem. org/) and the Women's Commission for Refugee Women and Children both have useful resources on the inclusion of women and children in disasters: (www.womenscommission. org/resources/index.cfm?limit=restype&limitID=4). The IASC also have a dedicated Gender Sub-Working Group with access to a variety of useful resources: (www.humanitarianreform.org/ Default.aspx?tabid=452#).

What are some of the specific issues confronting women and children in disaster situations? Each situation is unique but women and children, especially girls, can face:

- lack of protection, security and safety
- lack/loss of rights
- lack of power or representation (even though there may be greater numbers of women in emergency situations, for example if men have been called to fight, or have been killed)

- discrimination on the basis of gender is rife and may be culturally specific (for example through food distribution mechanisms)
- lack of gender awareness, or gender insensitivities (by agencies and organizations, for example regarding property rights or inheritance; or about remunerated work)
- lack of data or information about the situation of women or children
- assumptions (about needs or capabilities)
- lack of participation (often linked to misconceptions about abilities, or to gendered roles within communities)
- lack of priority (for example, of child protection programmes, education or maternal and child health)
- increased risk of violence, injury or death
- lack of access (for example to food programmes, fuel for cooking)
- specific health risks associated with disaster situations (including communicable diseases such as measles and diarrhoea; malnutrition; gender-based violence; rape and sexual violence).

There are also a vast number of resources that focus on children in disasters, including:

- The dedicated UN children's organization, UNICEF: (www.unicef.org/emerg/index.html)
- Save the Children UK: (www.savethechildren.org.uk/ assets/php/library.php?Topic=Emergencies)
- Plan International: (www.plan-international.org/resources/ publications/disasters/).

Older adults

Another group marginalized in disaster work with detrimental effects has been older adults. It is important to note that 'older adults' vary in age, role and responsibilities according to which communities they live in and, of course, their status is enormously affected by a disaster. HelpAge International has done a great deal of work in this area and has highlighted six common assumptions made by agencies and those involved in emergencies about older adults:

1. **The extended family and community will protect older people at all times** – this is rarely the case if the family have become separated, or are competing for scare resources.
2. **An agency will look after them** – there are no dedicated 'older adults' agencies, nor indeed international protection instruments; therefore they often slip through the net.
3. **They can be covered by general aid distributions** – not if they are unable to access distribution mechanisms or points for any number of reasons.
4. **They only have themselves to worry about** – often older adults are left to care for grandchildren and other members of the family as others flee, are injured, or die.
5. **They're waiting to be helped** – given the necessary support and structures, older adults have a wealth of experience, information and capabilities waiting to be used, and can be a useful community resource.
6. **They're too old to work** – again, older adults have experience and, given the right support, can be a fantastic supply for example regarding agricultural knowledge, cultural knowledge and history and location of natural resources.

There is also a useful list of resources and advice available in the joint publication from HelpAge Intentional and UNHCR:

● HelpAge International and UNHCR (n/d) *Older people in disasters and humanitarian crisis: Guidelines for best practice.* Uniform resource locator (URL): (www.helpage.org/Resources/ Manuals/main_content/1118336526-0-10/bpg.pdf).

People with disabilities
Another group that has been marginalized and excluded from aspects of planning, preparedness and responses to humanitarian emergencies is people with disabilities. They are, however, often

(Adapted from World Disaster Report 2007: 67).

disproportionately affected by the impacts of disasters, as a result of new impairments or disabilities, exacerbation of pre-existing conditions, and/or psychological traumas.

As with older adults, a number of assumptions are made about people with disabilities:

1. **They require specialist care** – this is in fact rarely the case. Many people with disabilities have been active members of the community prior to the disaster. As noted above, basic needs are the same for all, but it is how they are distributed that makes a difference. If family members, or adaptive devices and mobility aids are lost in the disaster, then previous levels of independence may be lost also. As long as they undertake fully inclusive programmes, humanitarian agencies can and should undertake to include disabled people in their programmes.
2. **Specialist care/adaptations are expensive** – as noted above, many adaptations can be undertaken in the initial phase with very little outlay and do not require expensive equipment or modifications.
3. **They will be covered by general aid distributions** – not if they are unable to access distribution mechanisms or points for any number of reasons. Therefore agencies must ensure distribution mechanisms are accessible – for example, the medium through which information is released (posters as well as via loud hailers or radios); ensuring water distribution points are accessible to mobility devices, etc.
4. **They cannot help other people** – on the contrary, disabled people may have skills that can be used in emergency and disaster situations and can work with rescue teams and members of their community to assist in location of other disabled people.
5. **They're waiting to be helped** – again, given the necessary support and structures, disabled people have a wealth of experience, information and capabilities that can be used within the affected communities, including in the recovery period when planning accessible reconstruction.

6. They're unable to work – some programmes (such as cash-for-work schemes) discriminate against people with disabilities, so humanitarian organizations should plan their programmes in an inclusive way, as, given the right encouragement and support, disabled people can participate in these programmes.

Disability has rarely been considered as a crosscutting issue in humanitarian responses – rather, disabled people are listed as a 'vulnerable group'. There is no specialist UN agency or IASC body dedicated to disability, or disability and humanitarian disasters. The recent UN Convention on the Rights of Persons with Disabilities (2008) may go some way to redress this and some donors are now making disability inclusion a criterion for programme funding. In order to fully achieve this, there will need to be better cooperation between humanitarian aid agencies, organizations specializing in disability issues, both on the national and international level and persons with disabilities, their families and communities as well as Disabled People's Organizations (DPOs) at all stages of disaster response, from planning to implementation. The creation of national and international guidelines will also facilitate this, though as yet none exists. There are, however, a number of useful resources, including from the Women's Commission, which provide practical guidance on inclusion, such as how to ensure refugee and IDP camps are accessible to people with disabilities and that they have full and equal access to the mainstream services that other refugees receive:

- Women's Commission (2008) *Disabilities among Refugees and Conflict-affected Populations:* resource kit for fieldworkers. (www.womenscommission.org/resources/index.cfm?limit=restype&limitID=4).

Minority groups (e.g. ethnic, cultural, linguistic, religious groups; pastoralists)

Minority groups, by their very definition, often exist at the margins of societies; sometimes this is out of choice, to protect lands or a lifestyle, other times it is because of persecution and necessity.

THINKING POINT

Because of their precarious living conditions and remote or marginal locations, minority groups are often very badly affected by disasters, especially those relating to the environment.

Minority groups are particularly vulnerable to the vagaries of climate change. Some minority groups are fighting conflicts, often with their own governments, to protect their way of life and environmental resources. As with other threatened and marginalized groups, they face:

- lack of protection, security and safety
- lack/loss of rights
- limited power or political representation
- discrimination, which may be culturally specific (for example of Roma)
- lack of awareness regarding minority rights
- lack of data or information about the situation of minority groups
- limited participation in wider social, cultural and political affairs
- lack of priority (due to relatively small numbers and often isolated living conditions)
- food insecurity (for example pastoralists who live in semi-nomadic conditions are at risk of drought, flooding and associated famines)
- poverty.

Ensuring full inclusion of minority groups means having a good understanding of local context, including the nature of the discrimination faced by minority groups, which goes beyond attitudinal issues to include structural and contextual aspects. This is particularly important in a disaster situation, where on the one hand agencies need to remain neutral and impartial to gain access to affected populations, but on the other, this may not only exacerbate existing tensions and discrimination of minorities, but also tacitly condone such behaviour if they are seen to be favouring one group over another.

For an extensive list of resources, please see the Minority Rights Group International website: www.minorityrights.org.

Refugees and Internally Displaced People (IDPs)

The Office of the United Nations High Commissioner for Refugees (UNHCR) was established on 14 December, 1950 by the United Nations General Assembly and takes the lead in refugee situations as mandated under the 1951 Refugee Convention and under the Global Cluster system. Over 150 countries have signed the convention and undertaken to protect refugees and not return them to a country where they may be persecuted (the principle of *non-refoulement*). The Convention was expanded in 1967 to include the protection of displaced people globally.

LEARNING POINT

Though UNHCR has taken on the protection of internally displaced people (IDPs) within its remit, IDPs do not have the protection of international refugee law and as yet there is no international legislation regarding care and protection of IDPs.

The UN has issued Guiding Principles on Internal Displacement; however, these are not an agreed legal principle but do offer a mechanism with which to argue for better safety, security and protection for IDPs. Though they have been incorporated into policy in a number of countries, including Angola, Burundi, Colombia, Georgia and Uganda, it has been argued that treating

IDPs differently from other citizens abdicates responsibility for them and in fact may restrict rights rather than improve them.

Accurate numbers of IDPs are hard to obtain, as it is very often their own states that are creating the protection problems for people in the first place. According to the Internal Displacement Monitoring Centre, by the end of 2006 the number of people internally displaced by conflict alone was estimated to be around 24.5 million people in 41 countries (IDMC: www.internal-displacement.org). There are IDPs in almost every continent of the world, though the vast majority are in Africa, including around 5.3 million people in Sudan. Women and children make up the majority of IDP populations (approximately 75–80 per cent), making protection issues even more essential.

Each refugee and IDP situation is different and many of the issues already highlighted above can be exacerbated by being in a refugee or IDP situation:

HAZARDS

- Lack of protection – especially the lack of international legislation for IDPs
- Lack of rights
- Loss of security and safety (IDPs in particular may be subject to policies and practices, particularly by their own governments, which have adverse effects on their security and status, as has happened in Darfur.)
- Limited representation (In fact, IDPs and refugees may be used as political pawns by opposing factions to highlight their cause, which may result in the situation being exaggerated or prolonged.)
- Discrimination on the basis of migrant status is rife across the world
- Specific risks associated with women and children who are refugees and IDPs (including health and gender-based violence)

- Lack of data or information about the situation of refugees and IDPs (especially protracted situations of displacement out of the eye of the media, donors or agencies)
- Assumptions (about needs or capabilities – or lack of these)
- Limited participation (often linked to misconceptions about abilities. This can lead to apathy and 'aid-dependency'.)
- Lack of priority (for example in education or maternal and child health programmes)
- Risk of violence, human rights abuses, injury or death (at any stage of flight to places of safety. Human rights abuses or attack may have been a strong contributing factor to displacement in the first place.)
- Lack of access (for example to water, food, healthcare and other essentials)
- Specific health risks associated with situations of displacement (including communicable diseases such as measles and diarrhoea; malnutrition; gender-based violence; rape and sexual violence)

The specific healthcare needs of refugees and IDPs at different points along the disaster cycle has been dealt with in Chapter 11. The list of UN organizations and other international and national NGOs providing healthcare at different points in this cycle is long and the reader is referred to resources outlined in other chapters. Refugees and IDPs, however, can be doubly or trebly discriminated against and marginalized, not only for their refugee or IDP status, but for many other reasons, such as on the basis of gender, HIV status, disability or minority group.

There are increasingly specific programmes to address some of these crosscutting issues. For example, Marie Stopes International works to improve sexual and reproductive health for refugees and IDPs: (www.mariestopes.org/Health_programmes/ Refugees_%5E_IDPs.aspx).

People living with HIV/AIDS

There are a number of diseases – such as AIDS, severe acute respiratory distress syndrome (SARS), avian influenza ('bird flu') – that are themselves viewed as a potential disaster and a threat to health and security (of borders, countries, people). The relationship between HIV and humanitarian emergencies is complex. In some countries HIV/AIDS has already caused situations akin to crisis, decimating populations and leaving children without parents, or being cared for by grandparents. This precarious situation is exacerbated by a disaster, leaving many adults and children especially vulnerable from loss of support networks, livelihoods and resources. During such times populations are more mobile, which may have an effect on modes of transmission. Moreover, as UNICEF has noted, emergency situations reduce the educational opportunities for children, depriving them of the chance to learn and understand about HIV and basic health services, leaving them yet more vulnerable. As noted above, children are already at increased risk of all forms of sexual exploitation in such situations.

Because of the effect on health service provision, there can be a long-term effect on the social, economic and political fabric of societies, exacerbating tensions and precipitating inequalities and potential conflicts. Inevitably, disasters and emergencies

CLINICAL CONSIDERATIONS

The prevalence of HIV can affect those tasked with assisting in situations of emergencies, but disasters can also affect health service provision and practice, such as blood screening and equipment sterilization techniques, as well as availability of treatment and public health measures to halt transmission.

can also exacerbate the situation of people living with HIV/AIDS in a number of ways, not least in the discriminatory way in which they may be treated in disaster situations.

Because of the complexity of the situation, the IASC initiated a dedicated task force on HIV in emergency settings to develop comprehensive guidance on the subject. Further information can be found at: www.humanitarianinfo.org/iasc/content/subsidi/tf_hiv/default.asp?bodyID=66&publish=0

The IASC produced *Guidelines for HIV and AIDS Interventions in Emergency Settings* in 2003, which provide recommendations on a wide range of areas and at different stages of response on prevention; basic care; protection of those affected; and workplace programmes for humanitarian workers. They can be downloaded from: www.who.int/hac/network/interagency/IASC_Guidlines_HIV_AIDS_in_Emergency_Settings.pdf

Finally, information collated by WHO, UNICEF, UNHCR and MSF regarding the provision of anti-retrovirals (ARVs) in emergency settings can be found at: www.aidsandemergencies.org/cms/index.php?option=com_content&task=view&id=35&Itemid=85

Summary

This chapter does not aim to be exhaustive or definitive – rather, it highlights some of the experiences of marginalization shared across diverse communities and peoples – of ignorance, exclusion, stigma and discrimination. It is important to note that resources, such as these listed here, are a starting point to provide the reader with some guides on ways to redress inequalities through actions that work to increase human rights and inclusion, but also to promote tolerance and understanding. This must be done by working with marginalized and vulnerable people, their families, friends, communities and their representative organizations to overcome barriers, increase awareness and advocacy. Successful inclusion cannot just be ticked off a checklist. Agencies must work together to promote best practices and to ensure that their own actions do not perpetuate exclusion and marginalization. Disaggregated information from assessments about social vulnerability can be shared so as to ensure those who potentially could slip through gaps are included in programmes. It is imperative that marginalized groups participate in all aspects of disaster planning, implementation and recovery – which may be for an extended duration. This means representation at every level. Finally, marginalized groups need to build alliances and share strengths between each other and use the opportunities that disasters can present to lobby for inclusion, equality and rights.

REFERENCES

Goodhand J. *Aiding Peace: the role of NGOs in armed conflict*. ITDG, Rugby, 2006.

IASC. *Guidelines for HIV/AIDS Interventions in Emergency Settings* (http://data.uraids.org/publications/External-Documents/iasc guidelines-emergency-se).

International Federation of Red Cross and Red Crescent Societies. *World Disaster Report*. IFRC, Geneva, 2007.

Kett M and Twigg J. Disability and disasters: towards an inclusive approach. In: *World Disaster Report 2007*. International Federation of the Red Cross and Red Crescent, Geneva, 2007.

Wells J. Older people and discrimination in crises. In: *World Disaster Report 2007*. International Federation of the Red Cross and Red Crescent, Geneva, 2007.

Healthcare in refugee populations

Aroop Mozumder

● Introduction

> **THINKING POINT**
>
> 'We need a humanitarian system that is able to respond reliably, effectively and efficiently across the full range of emergencies. Now more than ever, humanitarian aid must be the responsibility of all nations for the benefit of all nations'. Jan Egeland, UN Emergency Relief Coordinator.

Mass population movements, fleeing from either natural disasters or conflict zones, have become an increasingly important feature of the modern world. At the end of the 1990s, a US study on the demography of forced migration concluded that 30 million people were estimated to be internally displaced, with 23 million refugees, mostly as a result of conflict. **The difference between those internally displaced (IDPs), i.e. those remaining within a country of origin, and refugees who have crossed a border and are stateless, is important.** The UN High Commissioner for Refugees (UNHCR) has formal obligations for advocacy, responsibility and protection for refugees, but less so for those who are IDPs.

A mass population migration may be due to a natural disaster, such as an earthquake or tsunami, or a number of other factors, including conflict, deliberate targeting of populations or ethnic groups, increasing violence, food insecurity and fear. The response to the former event is often referred to as a humanitarian or disaster relief operation (HDRO). The latter, unfortunately increasingly common, is often termed a complex humanitarian emergency (CHE). In 2000, in a list of 24 countries meriting the term CHE, four countries (Afghanistan, Angola, North Korea and Sudan) each had over 3 million people affected.

A rapid refugee influx into an area can be regarded as a medical emergency affecting a whole population, with a requirement for rapid assessment of health needs, examination of key factors, basic investigations and 'treatment'; all of which must be instituted urgently, to minimize mortality and morbidity. In particular water, food, shelter, sanitation and healthcare are complementary factors that need to be addressed as a whole to support a refugee population; healthcare provision by itself is but one element. The international response to such events has been to set up refugee camps where a large number of agencies, both governmental, non-governmental (NGOs) and international (UN agencies) can deliver support to the population.

Over the past three decades there have been significant developments, with the emergence of evidence-based interventions, and wide acceptance of the principles of both needs assessment and priorities, often referred to as the **'Top Ten' priorities**. This chapter will give an overview of the evolution of health interventions for large displaced populations and describe the priorities for intervention. The immediate post-emergency phase, where health needs evolve into different priorities, will also be discussed.

● Today's reality of humanitarian interventions

Since the 1970s most developments in the health arena were normally curative, lacking norms and guidelines, with agencies working in isolation. However, this period did include the development of some significant advances, such as the management of severe malnutrition in therapeutic feeding centres (TFC), pioneered by Oxfam, Save the Children Fund-UK (SCF-UK) and Médecins Sans Frontières-France (MSF-France), with protocols used in a number of major emergencies.

From the early 1990s, there was more systematic use of data collection and surveillance and the growing awareness of the need for evidence based interventions and epidemiological concepts. Humanitarian assistance became a more specialist field with its own reference materials, policies and indicators.

More recently there has been acceptance of the need to include the views of the refugee community, with culturally acceptable care and increasing their active participation in relief programmes. However in the first phase of emergencies, a more standardized response has often been delivered in order to save life.

 THINKING POINT

The tension between regarding refugees as 'victims' with the delivery of a more 'paternalistic' model of care and regarding them as beneficiaries with a more inclusive approach remains an issue.

The SPHERE Project of 1998 was brought about by the coordinated activity of a number of established NGOs and the Red Cross and Red Crescent Movement, much influenced by the lessons identified from recent humanitarian crises. This brought considerations of accountability to beneficiaries and improved effectiveness in humanitarian aid delivery. It included the first statement of minimum standards of humanitarian relief in key areas such as water supply and healthcare, while linking these to fundamental human rights. These principles are now widely taught and adopted. In 2004 the revised SPHERE handbook developed and updated the themes of the first edition.

LEARNING POINT

Sphere Project 1998

'Meeting essential human needs and restoring life with dignity are core principles that should inform all humanitarian action. Through the Humanitarian Charter and Minimum Standards in Disaster Response, defined levels of service in water supply, sanitation, nutrition, food aid, shelter and site planning and healthcare are linked explicitly to fundamental human rights and humanitarian principles.'

Over 400 organizations in 80 countries contributed to the development of Minimum Standards and Key Indicators. **Overall, SPHERE is seen as a major advance in the development of standards in accountability and service delivery and is widely used.**

The first voluntary Code of Conduct was developed by the Red Cross movement and NGOs in 1994 (IFRCS, 1994). It sought to safeguard high standards of behaviour, maintain independence and promote effectiveness of disaster relief. In its 10 principles, the Code promoted respect for local culture, involvement of beneficiaries, building on local capacities and the impartial nature of aid. In 1999 nearly 150 agencies and 144 countries had signed up to the Code of Conduct, committing agencies to defined standards of behaviour.

● Priorities for intervention in disasters: the 'Top Ten' Priorities

L LEARNING POINTS

Top Ten Priorities
1. Initial needs assessment.
2. Measles vaccination and vitamin A supplementation in malnourished populations.
3. Water and sanitation.
4. Food and nutrition.
5. Shelter and site planning.
6. Healthcare in the emergency phase.
7. Communicable disease control.
8. Public health surveillance.
9. Human resources and training.
10. Coordination.
    To the top ten, an additional priority is often added:
11. Provision of security.

Refugees may have travelled great distances, normally by foot, before they reach a place of relative sanctuary. They may have been attacked, robbed, bereaved or wounded and often arrive in a camp exhausted, hungry, thirsty and traumatized. Their reaction may be that of anger, grief and apathy; in essence a modified bereavement reaction. It is important, however, not to assume that they are 'victims' who have lost all capacity for independent decision-making; they may be able to organize people into groups or village units, which will make the delivery of support much easier. There may also be village elders, interpreters or medically qualified individuals who will be of particular value.

The priorities for intervention for large displaced populations were developed for the seminal MSF Handbook, *Refugee*

Health: an approach to emergency situations (1997), which is now often adopted as the manual for those involved in humanitarian emergencies. The top ten priorities remain one of the most useful frameworks for those involved in emergency work. To these, an eleventh may be added, which is becoming of greater importance as conflict and complex emergencies are increasingly prevalent, that of provision of security. Security is now a basic parameter, providing 'humanitarian space' for other agencies, both governmental and NGO, to carry out their relief programmes.

1. Initial needs assessment in displaced populations

PEARL OF WISDOM

The importance of a rapid, comprehensive and concise needs assessment for displaced populations cannot be overemphasized. It is the first priority before any intervention is provided.

The data from a needs assessment may inform substantial operational planning in various NGO, UN, military and other organizations. The health needs assessment must be conducted within a few days. It will be constrained by the urgency to minimize mortality and morbidity, as well as the requirements of the tasking organization. The principle is to gather key facts on a range of important criteria, backed by evidence or reference, which can easily be provided to the HQ organization and upon which the main planning for the relief effort will be based.

Prior preparation, with climatic, environmental, geographical and area population detail before departing abroad is useful – much can be obtained from easily accessible databases. Shelter availability and quality, average number per shelter, diurnal variation in temperature, water availability and quality, and

Table 10.1 Health services assessment checklist (adapted from SPHERE)

Preparation	Information from host country database resources, maps, aerial photographs, health data.
Security and access	Natural and human hazards to security, presence of militias, access that humanitarian agencies have to the affected population, road access, proximity to ports and airports, communications. Food security.
Environmental factors	Climate, diurnal variation in temperature, rainfall.
Demography and social structure	Total population at risk (PAR), with proportion of children under 5 years. Identify groups at special risk, such as orphans, elderly, disabled/wounded. Ethnic mix and tensions, average household size.
Background health information	Identify pre-existing health problems in the area prior to the disaster, the epidemiology of pre-existing diseases in the refugee population, the potential new risks to health and potential for epidemic diseases. Nutritional status of PAR.
Mortality and morbidity rates	Calculate the crude mortality rate (CMR) and the under-5 mortality rate (U5MR).
Available resources	Assess current healthcare provision for locals and access for the refugee population. Status of local existing health resources, quality, bed numbers, skills of health staff, health information system, supply of medication and costs. Current health information data system.

sanitation facilities are fundamental factors, all of which need to be assessed and recorded (Table 10.1).

PEARL OF WISDOM

The camp environment is intimately related to the health outcomes of the resident population.

Access by road, availability of river or spring water, size of truck that can gain access and proximity to ports and airports, are also health determinants, albeit indirectly. Personnel resources and logistic considerations, such as the presence of specialist logistic NGOs or UN agencies need to be known. Communications, by telephone or internet can also make a vital difference in the organization of supplies and personnel.

Malnutrition prevalence can be assessed very crudely by observation (see Fig. 10.1), particularly of vulnerable groups such as children and the elderly – existing NGOs may have valuable data. The assessment of mortality rates, in particular the crude mortality rate (CMR) is fundamental to assessing the health of a population and in measuring the effectiveness of interventions. Morbidity rates for key diseases, such as malaria, acute respiratory infection or epidemic diseases may be recorded by medical NGOs. An understanding of prevalent disease is a core part of the needs assessment.

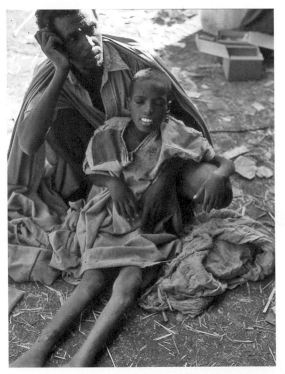

Fig. 10.1 Severe malnutrition with signs of Kwashiorkor in a 17-year-old Ethiopian girl during the famine in 1984.

The existing healthcare facilities: their type, quality, availability, appropriateness, diagnostic, laboratory and pharmaceutical support is required information, even if an NGO is providing these. Finally, brevity, accuracy and timeliness are key attributes of a good initial report. The urgency may allow only three working days or less to conduct the assessment. It should always be aimed at those who can act on the data: senior UN officials, the military chain of command, the host nation relief coordinator and senior NGO officials.

2. Measles immunization

High population density, particularly in rural populations displaced into camp settings, when linked with high levels of malnutrition, leads to extreme susceptibility to measles, one of the most contagious of diseases.

CLINICAL CONSIDERATIONS

Mass measles vaccination for children aged between 9 months and 15 years is the highest priority health intervention and cannot be delayed until other vaccines, or a more structured health service provision is available. This needs to be initiated within the first 10 days of a camp being established.

Logistic considerations, including the crucial importance of an effective cold chain, trained personnel and basics such as needles and syringes must be considered as a priority. The mortality rate from measles can exceed 2–21 per cent, following complications such as lobar pneumonia, diarrhoea, meningo-encephalitis and croup (Centers for Disease Control, 1992).

Very recently, due to the success of the WHO mass vaccination programmes, particularly in Africa, herd immunity against measles has markedly improved, such that the core importance of measles vaccine as a priority may be reduced in some areas of the world. However, in the presence of malnutrition, measles vaccination should always be considered as a priority unless there is definitive evidence to the contrary.

3. Water and sanitation

Lack of safe water, together with poor hygiene practices are a major cause of mortality and morbidity in displaced populations, particularly in the initial phases of a humanitarian emergency (see Fig. 10.2).

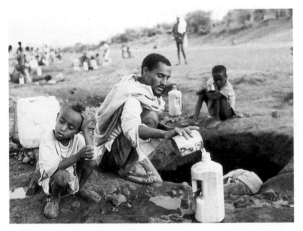

Fig. 10.2 Water taken from a riverbed in Sudan in 1985, adjacent to a large refugee camp for Tigrayan Ethiopians.

⚡ HAZARD

Epidemics of shigella dysentery and cholera have been recorded causing over 75 per cent of deaths in the initial emergency phase.

During the initial phase of the crisis the aim should be to provide 5 litres of water per person per day, as the bare minimum recommended by WHO for survival. However, this bare minimum provides only enough for food and drinking – hygiene is inevitably reduced, causing significant risk of transmissible disease. The aim must be to increase this to 15–20 litres of water per person per day. This will allow enough for washing, laundry and safer food preparation.

Sanitation, including safe disposal of human excreta is fundamental to the health of a displaced population. Attention to this issue is therefore an early and vital public health measure, which must take into account the expectations and cultural habits of the populations. These will include: separation of male from female latrines, knowing the distances people are prepared to walk to a latrine, hand-washing and privacy.

> ⚡ **HAZARD**
>
> Lack of respect for local culture may mean that sanitation facilities will not be properly used and excreta and waste may be left in the open, an obvious source of ill-health.

4. Food and nutrition

Protein-energy malnutrition is linked to vulnerability to disease, with measles being particularly important in causing mortality in the emergency phase. Nutritional assistance programmes are therefore an important priority to reduce mortality in any displaced population. WHO recommends the minimum food ration of 2100 Kcal per person per day; this has remained the basic aim of nutritional programmes for some decades, with an appropriate nutrient balance. Health staffs are usually involved in nutritional assessment, management and selective feeding of those with more serious malnutrition and advising other agencies on the suitability of the rations delivered. The general ration may be made up of purchased rations in the local markets, if available, or the introduction of substantial amounts of food aid from major donors. The ration distribution system needs to be fair and equitable. Care needs to be taken that the local economy is not disrupted, either by flooding the market with cheap donated grain, or driving up prices by bulk purchase such that the locals cannot afford market produce. Either case can lead to major friction with the host community. The nutritional status of a population is usually extrapolated from assessment of children under 5 years. Weight for Height (WHF), as a percentage against internationally agreed child growth norms, is widely accepted as the most sensitive and accurate measure of nutritional status (Young and Jaspers, 1995).

Selective feeding programmes are normally required for the proportion of children with acute malnutrition, before or even despite a reasonable overall ration for the population. Therapeutic Feeding Centres (TFC) are heavily resource intensive (see Fig. 10.3). They are in-patient facilities, where children are admitted, normally with their mother or elder sibling, to correct dehydration, and to treat severe malnutrition and infections. Such children are seriously ill, with a high mortality. They are often apathetic and need to be encouraged to take food and may suffer other complications such as hypothermia, even in tropical climates. They need feeding at regular intervals, often through the night in the most acute cases. High energy milk is often supplemented by vitamin A, antibiotics and treatment of intestinal parasites. In younger infants, breast feeding should

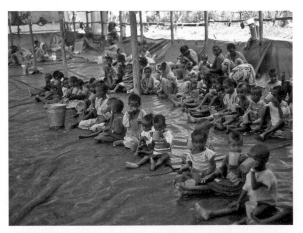

Fig. 10.3 A therapeutic feeding centre in Ethiopia in 1985 operated by SCF-UK.

continue, if the mother is present. Supplementary feeding is for those children with a less acute, although still serious malnutrition measure, in terms of percentage WFH. Normally children attend as 'out-patients' for a few hours of additional feeding. They are also given a supplementary ration to take home, so that other members of the family may benefit.

Finally, there needs to be an awareness of micronutrient deficiencies in acute emergency situations. Xerophthalmia (vitamin A deficiency), pellagra (vitamin B3 deficiency), scurvy (vitamin C deficiency), anaemia (iron deficiency) and goitre (iodine deficiency) are particularly common, although a number of other conditions may be seen.

5. Shelter and site planning

HAZARD

Effective shelter is of obvious health benefit. Overcrowding, when combined with poor hygiene, is conducive to the transmission of major outbreaks of disease such as shigella dysentery and cholera.

The principles are that: a camp must have a limited population density and be in family groups per shelter, traditional village structures should be replicated as far as possible, and access to essential facilities, such as water and latrines, must be reasonable.

6. Healthcare in the emergency phase

The unique features of an acute emergency, of high morbidity, high levels of mental stressors and comparatively easy access to healthcare, often leads to unexpectedly large demand, where many may have self-limiting disease. **Adequate triage:** the ability to screen rapidly, assess and treat the more serious cases, is an important requirement for any health system. The accepted form of healthcare facilities, pioneered by MSF and

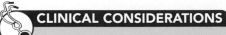

CLINICAL CONSIDERATIONS

It is important to realise that in the vast majority of refugee emergencies, the main causes of mortality are due to four disease groups: diarrhoeal diseases, respiratory infections, malaria and measles, normally complicated by underlying malnutrition. The mainstay of medical care is therefore to be able to diagnose and treat the majority of illness, using simple diagnostic and treatment protocols (SPHERE-based), that can be taught to local and other health workers.

other NGOs are based on the four levels outlined in the following Learning Points box:

LEARNING POINTS

Key Levels of Healthcare

1. Basic care and screening from a local home visitor from the refugee population, for every 500 people.
2. A small health post with a trained health worker, with a limited dispensary, working to agreed protocols for common diseases, for up to 5000 people.
3. A more central health centre, with a doctor and nurses, with limited in-patient facility, for every 30000 people. This facility is capable of seeing referrals from health posts, treating more complex cases, providing simple surgical procedures and uncomplicated obstetric and midwifery care. This will have simple laboratory services, such as malaria blood film screening and microscopy for parasites. The single doctor may only have time to provide guidance on preventive medicine policy, to undertake training and to see complex cases.
4. A referral hospital facility, which can carry out emergency surgery, treatment of wounds, complex obstetric care and a referral laboratory.

WHO have developed emergency health kits (WHO, 1995), suitable for a displaced population emergency situation, to treat a population of 10000 for 3 months with protocol-based medications and dressings. These have been in use worldwide for many years. The importance of providing reproductive health services and mental health services is increasingly recognized as being valuable, early in an emergency, and should not be forgotten.

7. Communicable disease control

As described, the four major causes of death in many mass displaced person settings, particularly when associated with malnutrition may cause 60–90 per cent of all deaths. In addition, typhoid, meningococcal meningitis, yellow fever, typhus, plague, dengue, leishmaniasis, polio and viral hepatitis often cause major outbreaks. In terms of more chronic disease, TB, particularly when multi-drug resistant, and HIV/AIDS can be a serious problem.

Preparing and planning for epidemics, which will almost invariably occur, requires good background health intelligence. When an outbreak arises, the cases must initially be confirmed. This requires proper history taking and examination of initial cases, followed by laboratory confirmation if at all possible. If confirmed, successive cases may be diagnosed based on standardized field definitions, such as those from SPHERE. Control of any outbreak will include: finding and minimizing the sources, interrupting transmission of disease, such as vector control measures in malaria, and the protection of susceptible groups. Cooperation with the local Ministry of Health protocols and WHO reporting systems is important.

Diarrhoeal diseases are a principal cause of morbidity and mortality in refugee situations. *Shigella*, rotavirus, cholera and *Escherichia coli* are significant pathogens. Bloody diarrhoea with fever is a strong indication that *Shigella* is present, which needs laboratory confirmation. Adequate oral rehydration therapy (ORT) networks and trained workers, attention to camp and personal hygiene, clean water supply, adequate food rations and the promotion of breast-feeding for infants are key control measures. Successful ORT needs effort; not all refugee populations or health workers are convinced of its efficacy.

Acute watery diarrhoea, particularly when arising in patients over 5 years, resulting in severe dehydration, must be presumed to be cholera. A cholera outbreak in any camp consumes significant resources and must be planned for.

> **THINKING POINT**
>
> Cholera can have a case fatality rate of up to 50 per cent without treatment but, with proper management, it can be well under 2 per cent.

Acute respiratory infections (ARIs) may be defined as any case of fever, cough and rapid respiratory rate. It is relatively easy to diagnose by trained health workers by finding the abnormal breath sounds of lobar pneumonia. Many ARIs are upper respiratory and more mild, but serious disease is common in conditions of overcrowding, particularly when associated with poor shelter, wet climatic conditions and malnutrition. The cause is normally *Streptococcus pneumoniae* and *Haemophilus influenzae*, both of which can be treated with oral antibiotics in most cases. Case finding, use of field definitions and adequate training for health workers is important in controlling ARIs.

Malaria can be a major problem, particularly with refugees who have migrated to an area of higher endemicity. Malaria protection is based on controlling the vector: by minimizing standing water, larvicide spraying, use of permethrin-impregnated mosquito nets (where resources permit) and periodic spraying of shelters. Chemoprophylaxis is a subject of debate but, in some emergencies, administration to malnourished children and pregnant women has been considered.

8. Public health surveillance

Information is vital in measuring effectiveness of a response. This must be systematically collected, standardized for collation, appropriate and acceptable to the Ministry of Health, acceptable to those affected, and regular and timely enough to be useful. It is important to be consistent, rapid, repeatable, rather than always absolutely exact. Many NGOs, donor organizations and other international organizations may base their response on the available health data; it is therefore a core requirement. Key information includes the CMR, morbidity from key diseases and nutritional surveillance data.

9. Human resources and training

Most NGOs responding to a relief programme will tend to send a small group of ex-patriots, who will support their own locally recruited resident personnel who may have worked in the country for some years. An intervention programme will often mean a rapid recruitment of a significant number of local staff, with a variety of logistic, medical engineering or administrative skills. Western military forces may be one of the few groups that are relatively self-sufficient in terms of manpower; however, even they are increasingly recruiting interpreters and other key staff. Expatriate staff are increasingly required to have appropriate training and supervision when they deploy to an emergency. This effectively means that elements of 'Clinical Governance' and increased accountability are of greater importance and are welcome features of relief programmes.

10. Coordination

Coordination by the various agencies responding to a common humanitarian goal does in theory sound a simple proposition. In past decades, however, this has sometimes been problematic and resulted in major system failings. The performance of the international community following the genocide in Rwanda provides one example. There have, however, been some recent improvements in inter-agency cooperation. A well coordinated relief effort has a number of features: leadership, normally from a UN agency working closely with the host government, an effective coordinating body with some lower level executive authority, agreed inter-agency priorities and rationalization of activity such that 'economies of scale' can be achieved. Where donor organizations, international military forces and other international organizations are present, it is useful for them to have a seat at coordination meetings. This, of course, may create tensions in some areas, but has also been seen to work effectively.

11. Provision of security

Although not always considered core to the 'Top Ten' priorities for assistance to large displaced populations, the provision of adequate security is fundamental to all other public health and welfare interventions. The control of violence between tribes or ethnic groups, gender violence and fear within a displaced community, are immensely harmful to population health and well-being. The imposition of security can occur from a range of actors: the host population police or army, a NATO, UN or other western peacekeeping force, a more local military force, such as one from the African Union, or even militia within the refugee population themselves.

● Participants in a major refugee emergency

A refugee crisis can result in a confusing number of organizations arriving, each with their own mandates and priorities. The leadership and coordination will normally come from a senior UN representative, such as the representative of the UN High Commissioner for Refugees (UNHCR) or UN Office for the Coordination of Humanitarian Affairs (UNOCHA). Often the host nation may have a senior representative of their Interior Ministry or a Relief Commissioner, who will be a co-chair at meetings with the UN representative. Alongside these may be field officers from the major donor nations, such as from the UK Department for International Development (DFID) or the US Agency for International Development (USAID). Other major UN organizations, such as the World Food Programme (WFP), UNICEF and WHO, will be supporting their specialist areas of food delivery, vaccines and health policy respectively.

NGOs, of which several may be present in any humanitarian emergency, are private organizations, which raise funds from the public but are increasingly funded by governments for specific programmes. For example in the UK, most NGOs have charitable status and may bid for funds from DFID for a specific intervention programme, as well as direct appeals through the media to the public for funds. NGOs have their own mandates, which enable them to gain expertise in a particular field of relief work. Many, such as Oxfam, SCF, MSF and Merlin have international reputations for high quality relief programmes. However, when a number of NGOs and other agencies arrive in a disaster situation, significant effort is required to provide a coherent, balanced and appropriate response.

Host nation security and police forces will normally have controls and checkpoints of entry and exit to a camp. Their senior officials may be part of the coordination meetings. Lastly, there is an increasing tendency for governments, particularly in the West, to deploy military forces to disaster or CHE areas. In particular, airlift, logistic support, engineering and medical support are capabilities often deployed.

● The post-emergency phase

The post-emergency phase, normally considered to have started when the core priorities have been addressed, with some population stability and a reduction in the CMR to below 1 in 10 000 per day, is an opportunity to address broader health-related activities. These include:

- **The introduction of the WHO Extended Programme for Immunization (EPI)**, which normally includes: diphtheria, pertussis, polio, measles, tetanus and BCG.

- **Maternal and child health clinics (MCH).** Reproductive healthcare normally includes ante-natal, delivery and post-natal care, family planning, STD and HIV/AIDS care and supporting victims of sexual violence. Child healthcare includes basic curative care for common diseases as well as the EPI and growth monitoring and health promotion activity.
- **A tuberculosis treatment programme**, which involves regular treatment and monitoring over a period of several months, including directly observed treatment clinics (DOTS), needs relative population stability. When to start such programmes may present ethical dilemmas: the population may not be stable enough to start such a programme, the quality of treatment may be better than that received by the host population, with poor compliance, resistance, HIV/TB prevalence and poor administration being considerations.
- **Mental health programmes** are often regarded as a lower priority in the acute phase of a refugee emergency, where the focus is on the immediate physical needs. However, it is vital to address the psychosocial needs as soon as possible. Part of the population, particularly those significantly traumatized, may be unable to make use of food distribution and healthcare; if they are mothers, their children are especially vulnerable. How best to address this need remains a controversial area; western style counselling has not been shown to be effective, with more culturally appropriate social support having some advantages.

The post-emergency phase may present different challenges. **There is the risk of dependency and permanency within a camp, which will be a key concern of the host government.** In particular increasing economic activity from refugees, from trading donated goods, manufacturing and labour, may have a significant impact on the local economy and employment. For this reason, repatriation to the original country is always preferred as an outcome, once conditions there have improved.

Rwanda 1994

Quality and programme evaluation have been increasingly important themes since the mid-1990s, particularly since the evaluation of the relief operation to Rwanda in 1994 by the UK-based Overseas Development Institute (ODI), which in 1995 published a *Joint Evaluation of Emergency Assistance to Rwanda*. Until then there was a widespread view, both among aid workers and the general public, that 'humanitarian workers were always doing good'. The increase in media exposure and scrutiny, in particular to the prolonged Rwanda emergency changed this view. The ODI report stated that 100 000 avoidable deaths could be attributed to the poor performance of the relief agencies. Lack of standards, weak accountability and poor coordination were principle factors. The Report also noted failures in a number of key areas: lack of policy coherence, lack of coordination between UN and humanitarian agencies as well as government teams and military contingents, poor quality healthcare from many NGOs and inadequate accountability of agencies and their inability to assess their impact. It was partly due to these failures that the established NGOs and the Red Cross movement developed standards of behaviour and performance, which led to the Code of Conduct, SPHERE and significant quality improvements.

Summary

There has been considerable progress in the evidence base for the health management of a major humanitarian disaster, whether naturally caused or due to conflict. Initial assessment and priorities for intervention are well established, with increasing cooperation and integration of the relief effort becoming evident, although progress is still required. Humanitarian aid, however, remains dominated by the western model of aid delivery, although other systems, for example bilateral systems from Russia and China, also exist. The views of the recipients of aid, the refugees, are only comparatively recently being taken into account.

The need for all health workers in this area to be adequately trained in this emerging medical specialty, with an understanding of both the requirements at field level and a higher strategic appreciation of how an aid effort is coordinated and delivered are key skills, which can significantly improve healthcare delivery to some of the world's most vulnerable people.

REFERENCES AND FURTHER READING

References

Centers for Disease Control. Famine affected, refugee, and displaced populations: Recommendations for public health issues. *MMWR* 1992; **41** (RR-13): 1–76.

International Federation of Red Cross and Red Crescent Societies. *Code of Conduct for the International Red Cross and Red Crescent Movement and NGOs in Disaster Relief*. Geneva, 1994. Available at: http:/www.ifrc.org/publicat/conduct/ (Accessed: 24 August 2008).

Médecins Sans Frontières. *Refugee Health: an approach to emergency situations*. Macmillan Education, London, 1997.

WHO. *The New Emergency Health Kit*. World Health Organization, Geneva, 1990.

Young H and Jaspars S. *Nutrition Matters*. Intermediate Technology Publications, London, 1995.

Further reading

Healing TD, Drysdale SF, Black ME *et al*. Monitoring health in the war affected areas of the former Yugoslavia 1992–93. *European Journal of Public Health* 1996; **6**: 245–51.

Heymann D. (ed.) *Control of Communicable Diseases in Man*. (18th Edition). American Public Health Association Press, 2005.

Mahoney P and Ryan J. (eds) *Conflict and Catastrophe Medicine: a practical guide*. Springer Verlag, New York, 2009.

Simmonds S, Vaughan P and Gunn W. *Refugee Community Health Care*. Oxford Medical Publications, Oxford, 1983.

The SPHERE Project. *Humanitarian Charter and Minimum Standards in Disaster Response*. (2nd Edition). SPHERE, 2004. Available at: www.sphereproject.org (Accessed: 24 August 2008).

11 The realities of war

Jonathan Kaplan, an anonymous military author and Laith K. Alrubaiy

● Introduction

War is a human disaster with many far-reaching consequences for those whose lives it touches. For some war is a catastrophe that descends upon them, while others immerse themselves in it voluntarily, alongside the combatants or, with a compulsion to address its destructive aftermath. Each individual's perception of the conflict about them will be unique so this chapter aims to give some brief insights into the realities of war from the perspectives of a surgeon, a soldier and a medical student in times of conflict. Jonathan Kaplan's experiences, operating under fire in many of the world's recent conflicts, are evocatively recorded in his books *The Dressing Station* and *Contact Wounds*. Our military author is a doctor with experience, in and out of uniform, of wars around the globe and writes here, out of necessity, anonymously. Laith Alrubaiy was a medical student at the time of the US-led invasion of Iraq and learned the medical arts amidst its human consequences.

Going to war

Jonathan Kaplan

A humanitarian organization is sending you to work in a war zone. You have been briefed on the aim of your deployment, your organization's mission-concept and its organizational structure in the field. There will have been information on security, health issues and speaking to the media; NGOs are understandably particular about image management in the fierce competition for donor attention. Background data on regional politics, conflict history and cultural conditions – of varying usefulness – may have been provided. However, the assumption is that the professional and personal resources you'll be taking along to cope with the conditions you will face, are all your own.

Your relevant prior experience will probably have been of peacetime hospital work. Patients arriving in the Emergency Department receive their injuries in some known place: at work, in the street, a transport accident, on a building site. They're tended to by others – passers-by, first-aiders or paramedics – then carried by ambulance to the expected environs of a hospital and, depending on the level of urgency, brought or rushed through to the doctor. Step by step, they've taken on the role of being a patient. The same process – being hit, tended by a medic, transferred to the aid post, evacuated to a surgical facility – is the rule for military wounded in war: the concept of being cared for, of putting oneself in the hands of others, of being a casualty with an injured person's right to treatment.

The casualties you'll be treating are often without those rights. Their communities may have been displaced, social structures wrecked. Some might bear arms, though generally they are victims, guilty simply of trying to survive a cataclysm that has overwhelmed their lives, homes and families. Now they have been wounded, struck down, with all the fear of sudden mortality. The transfer to your place of care may have been a dash in a vehicle under fire or a journey in a blanket-litter over mountains, enduring pain and cold and uncertainty. Sometimes they've been shot just round the corner, run to your location on someone's back with screams and panic and they're dumped at your feet in clothes that stink of smoke and brick-dust, unhinged by terror or the madness of gunfire. And you, yanked abruptly from sleep, overwhelmed by numbers and blood, may be in little better shape yourself.

That shock is something to get over. Advanced Trauma Life Support (ATLS®) training helps, as does the application of a rigorous triage system, but no matter how well you memorize the triage sieve card (see Fig. 1.1) – and it's been made as simple as possible, the better to retain it under pressure – the initial response, the first and second and possibly third time you are placed in this unforgiving arena, is one of confusion: where is this blood coming from? why is the patient collapsed? what is this unrecognizable mess, that screaming, those nerve-wracking explosions?

● The doctor under fire

THINKING POINT

Formal wars conducted between nations are rare. Instead they are increasingly unstructured, their stated goals – 'war on terror' – often nebulous. Most conflict situations you will find yourself in are due to the collapse of societies: civil war, insurgencies, freelance militia groups indistinguishable from banditry.

Shells and bullets tend to fly randomly, though it is sadly the case that humanitarian workers are increasingly shot at intentionally. Becoming a prospective target tends to cloud your judgement. Besides the fear, there's nothing lonelier than being under fire; being abandoned by your assistants in the middle of surgery as they run for cover, compounds the sense of helplessness. Your medical training has accustomed you to interpret data – history, examination findings, options for treatment – and act on these, but here too many factors are unknowable, the computations for a right decision intolerably complex, for on them depends the survival not only of your patient but of yourself.

Judging whether you should stay or run is usually out of your hands; most NGOs have strict procedures for minimizing risk to their personnel and will evacuate you at the first sign of real danger. But if the decision is yours, you might regard it as an extension of triage. Your aim is to obtain the best outcome for the greatest number, rather than one individual patient, who may indeed have to be put aside to continue to suffer, or even placed in the 'expectant' category of those who are denied definitive care because they are not expected to live. By similar criteria, there comes a point when the danger of your physical position in the line of fire exceeds any possible benefit. As in triage management, you do not expend all available resources on the care of a single casualty.

> **PEARL OF WISDOM**
>
> You, as a doctor, are a most vital asset. Dead, you are useless; wounded, a liability.

Don't underestimate how fatigue diminishes your ability to think. Exhaustion leads to numbness and fatalism. The absence of colleagues with whom to share the hard responsibility of making clinical choices wears you down, as does immersion in war itself, with its relentless stupidity and violence. The illusion that surgical miracles can be achieved through good intentions alone is soon dispelled; a lack of resources means that patients die of conditions or complications that would be easily treatable in your hospital back home and every loss diminishes your sense of the worth of what you are doing. It is when you are faced with a rush of casualties – or the realization that no matter how many you treat, more will be coming – that you are most likely to feel overwhelmed and unable to cope. But in reality what you are facing is a single problem: how to help the person in front of you.

● Treating war-wounded

It is experience that convinces you that you can intervene effectively, that you are making a difference. Resuscitative

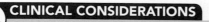

CLINICAL CONSIDERATIONS

The steps are simple. Remember the triage card. Count those breaths yourself. That leads you automatically to consider what will kill your patient fastest: blocked airway, breathing problems (tension or 'open' – big hole in the chest – pneumothorax, massive haemothorax, flail chest). Fragment and bullet injuries can kill through massive blood loss and this may be the first and most obvious problem to address. So as you measure the pulse you think of circulation, of external and hidden haemorrhage, including cardiac tamponade, bleeding into the chest and abdomen and pelvis, as well as blood loss from long bone fractures. And as you think, you are performing the resuscitation.

physiology is relatively basic: adequate oxygenation via a functional airway and breathing mechanism, plus a circulating volume with sufficient oxygen-carrying capacity to perfuse vital organs, should maintain life. You secure the airway by some form of intubation, start intravenous infusion and place intercostal drains to allow effective ventilation. Emergency surgery – correcting cardiac tamponade, stopping major haemorrhage, controlling contamination from gut perforation or meningeal tear – can then follow. These are damage-limitation procedures, with the intention that definitive surgery will be carried out when proper expertise and resources are available.

Be reassured, it is most unlikely that you will find yourself in so dire a situation: treating casualties single-handed, on or near a front line, with minimal resources and shells falling around you. If you do, then the very extremity of your situation will limit what you can achieve. Patients reach you with massive multi-system injuries that require the most intensive intervention, in precisely the situation where you are least able to give it. You could be working as a doctor in a besieged town, with no facilities for evacuation of wounded. You may not be directly under fire, but the degree of isolation is similar. Severely wounded patients may not survive the process of getting to you, or if they do, may have injuries that are not treatable with the means available. All you can do is the best you can. Remember the aim of Disaster Medicine intervention – to reduce *excess* morbidity and mortality – and the simple equation that anything you are doing to reduce the suffering of even one person alleviates in some degree the sum of the suffering of all.

● Getting yourself home

Working in a war zone requires a fairly explicit set of intellectual adjustments, for which your medical training will largely have prepared you: to face problems and challenges, formulate an approach, modify your response according to the outcome and apply your new knowledge. Despite the fatigue and the frustrations, the experience can be extraordinarily constructive. It is coming home, to the ordered demands of your previous existence, that presents the greatest emotional shock. The more intense the experience you have been through, the more extreme the readjustment. Exposure to war is a brutalizing experience that may affect, for a while at least, your own ability to reconnect with those around you. You will certainly have made discoveries about the limitations of your abilities and the consequences of your actions; as a surgeon, you might have encountered someone like a water engineer who, by bringing clean water to an IDP (Internally Displaced Persons) camp, will have saved more lives than you could if you operated non-stop for the next fifty years. In your more introspective moments you may judge your personal contribution to have been marginal, a poor application of resources. But humility and compassion are the only antidotes to war's destructive idiocy. The benefit you'll have brought to others is incalculable and your life will be changed forever.

FURTHER READING

Giannou C. *Besieged: A Doctor's Story of Life and Death in Beirut*. Bloomsbury, London, 1991.

Hedges C. *War is a Force That Gives Us Meaning*. Anchor Books, New York, 2003.

Kaplan J. *Contact Wounds: a war surgeon's education*. Picador, London, 2005.

Kaplan J. *The Dressing Station: a surgeon's odyssey*. Picador, London, 2001.

Mahoney PF, Ryan JM, Brooks AJ and Schwab CW. (eds) *Ballistic Trauma: a practical guide*. (2nd Edition). Springer-Verlag, London, 2004.

Van Rooyen M, Kirsch T, Clem K and Holliman CJ. (eds) *Emergent Field Medicine*. McGraw Hill, New York, 2002.

Helmand

Anonymous

It's that usual military thing, a couple of hundred squaddies, assorted beret colours and cap badges, assembled on the Helmand parade ground unnecessarily long in advance of the ceremony. Not all men...there's a sprinkling of women too. How many more weeks have I got out here? Minutes standing around in groups before being asked to 'form up' on three sides of a square, whilst the sergeant major struts around, making sure that this evolution, of all evolutions, will proceed to plan. Baking heat, bright sunshine, light breeze stirring up the dust. Several padres, distinguished by the colourful religious sashes worn over their combat fatigues, stand in a huddle, exchanging small talk before being awkwardly joined by a Commanding

Officer or two. Finally it's time to start, with the group marching out to the dais...but then Commanding Officers never could march and the padres don't even try, shuffling along clutching their sashes and Bibles to their bellies.

Three sides of the square are brought to attention, relieved of the tedium of inactivity. A padre begins and over the tannoy we hear details of the two men who died in the explosion three days previously. A couple of mates have been chosen to march out and read tributes...one of the men had a lively love life...the other played guitar...both were great blokes. Somehow the wankers never get killed. Family back home...widows, children without fathers, parents without sons. The Commanding Officer reads a lesson from the Bible, the padre completes the religious ceremony and then there's the minute's silence, ominously ushered in and out with a retort from one of the two field guns set up in the corners of the parade square. Then a recording of the last post...and even as this is being played there's the throb of helicopter rotors overhead: a Chinook. The MERT, Medical Emergency Response Team, helicopter is arcing into the landing site on the other side of Camp Bastion and every man and woman's thoughts on that damnable concrete square in that far off god-forsaken country are drawn to the severely injured soldiers contained within, being delivered to the hospital.

Military medicine in the UK is 'enjoying' a renaissance: medical 'fly-on-the wall' soap operas of resuscitations at Camp Bastion are suddenly the fodder of prime-time television and glossy weekend broadsheet magazines. Senior military doctors are now feted at international conferences, eager to share their latest knowledge of the best resuscitation fluid regimens and innovative use of blood transfusion products. But this has not come lightly... it is the legacy of what has become a brutal, grinding conflict with no end in sight. Forward Operating Bases ringed with hidden enemy IEDs (improvised explosive devices) ready to catch the unwary patrol. For all the extra armour clad to the sides and bellies of the patrol vehicles, there are yet bigger explosive devices attached to the buried pressure-plate initiators.

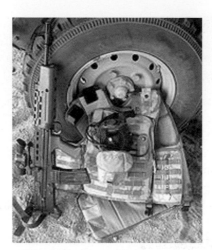

Fig. 11.1 Osprey combat body armour.

Combat body armour: in the Falklands War no body armour was worn; the Royal Marines even dispensed with the helmets issued in favour of the comfort of the signature 'green beret'. But since then there's been progress – military medical researchers beetling away in the depths of laboratories and blast chambers, firing bullets into gelatine blocks and detonating explosions in order to develop protection for our soldiers against the ravages of war (Fig. 11.1). The result? A blast and bullet protective helmet combined with a body armour protecting chest and abdomen... and it's effective. Suddenly those central penetrating injuries which formerly carried such high mortality are prevented. This is not, however, without a cost: the armour affords little protection to limb and face. Those soldiers who would previously have died of their central wounds are now surviving, but with the burden of amputations of one, two, three and even four limbs and perhaps severe facial blast injury.

With necessity being the mother of invention, the challenges posed by the Afghan Conflict have led to considerable development in UK military medicine.

The military are now at the forefront of developing new fluid resuscitation protocols, drawn from a combination of scientific

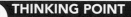

THINKING POINT

For every casualty reported in the UK media there is a multiplier of three or four with such a severe spectrum of injury. For these soldiers, no more the dream of sporting prowess or a special forces career. Instead the burden of lifelong disability and pain. Furthermore the body armour has been criticized for being too heavy and limiting mobility. Due to the weight, personnel are more likely to be vehicle borne, increasing vulnerability to IED attack.

HAZARD

It has been realized that massive haemorrhage is the most common cause of **preventable** death of a soldier in war. This has led to the abandonment of the civilian *Advanced Trauma Life Support* doctrine of ABCDE prioritization in favour of an approach emphasizing the prevention of massive haemorrhage by pressure bandage, tourniquet and haemostatic dressings (*Quick Clot* or *Hemcon*).

endeavour in UK military medicine research establishments and real experience in the field with multiply-injured casualties. The Medical Emergency Response Team (MERT) helicopter is able, within minutes, to take advanced life support virtually to the point of wounding and then effect evacuation to the hospital in Camp Bastion where life and limb-saving surgery can take place. For the injured British serviceman this will typically be followed by evacuation to the UK, usually within 24 hours of injury and many a wounded soldier, losing consciousness as a victim of an IED in the deserts of Helmand, will next wake up in a hospital in Selly Oak, Birmingham. Enemy forces, Afghan government security forces and Afghan civilians also have access, for life, limb and sight-threatening

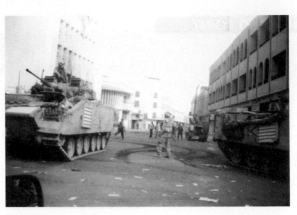

Fig. 11.2 British Soldiers in Basra.

injuries, to the MERT and treatment at Bastion, but are then passed on to other Afghan health facilities.

The war in Afghanistan shows no sign of abating and UK servicemen and women are likely to be needed for several more years at least (Fig. 11.2). In support of this mission, military medical services will be required, made up from both regular and reserve forces personnel. Regular doctors undergo regular roulement through the operational hospitals whilst the Territorial Army medical services, once a flabby social and dining club with only a remote chance of operational deployment are now suddenly front line, with an expectation if not obligation to undertake overseas operational roles. Resuscitation...primary surgery...evacuation...and the injuries keep coming, heralded by the throb of the MERT's rotors over the parched Helmand Desert.

Life in war

Laith Alrubaiy

War is a state of open, armed, often prolonged conflict carried on between nations, states, or parties. It is a mixture of the

CASE STUDY

The first Gulf War

As other countries started to move towards the new millennium and Iraq began to heal its wounds from the 8 year Iraqi–Iranian war, the Gulf War started as a result of the Iraqi invasion of Kuwait. The situation started with international economic sanctions in 1990. These sanctions completely isolated Iraq from the rest of the world. They prevented food, fuel and medicines from reaching the besieged country areas. Shortly afterwards, the war started. The Iraqi army burned the oil wells in Kuwait and poured the oil into the Arab Gulf. Toxic chemicals from the damaged oil facilities contributed to water pollution. The sky was clouded with black from the burned oil wells and it rained black rain in Basra at that time. We had to use the shower room as a shelter. For that reason, we put many sand bags on the roof to protect us from bombs and shrapnel and we stripped the window glass to prevent its shattering into pieces.

Whenever there was a raid all lights had to be turned off and small candles were used instead, as a procedure to elude the striking airplanes. Due to shortage of water, people had to collect rain water and let it settle before drinking it. I saw many children die in hospitals because of acute gastroenteritis attacks. The war damaged the drug stores and what was left was looted. Beds, chairs and medical equipment were stolen. Lack of electricity was one of the main problems in hospitals. Electricity was interrupted and the standby generators couldn't work for more than a few hours during the day. The water supply to hospitals was not enough and many patients had to bring their own bottles to drink water or wash their hands. Without electricity, medical staff could not monitor vital signs of the patients. Vaccines and some medicines that had to be kept at low temperatures could not be safely used. Drugs were sold without any supervision and most of them were expired due to lack of proper storage conditions.

The serious civilian casualties added growing pressure on hospitals and health workers. Staff worked extremely long hours in unimaginable circumstances and some vital surgical and medical supplies ran short. Gasoline shortages were a constant. Long queues of up to 10 km were not uncommon and people had to wait for as long as 8 hours to fill their cars. Thus, a flourishing black market for selling petrol appeared. Due to constant electricity cuts, Iraqis were forced to use wood to cook and warm their homes during the winter months. This had led to an increase in burn victims. Most of the time the rooms were very small and there was not good ventilation, which led to many cases of gas poisoning being seen in hospitals.

psychological, social, educational, humanitarian and other harmful consequences of human beings' desire to dominate. To understand Disaster Medicine, a doctor should be aware of the quality of life and the implications of wars. I have lived through two big wars. The Iraqi-Iranian war (1980–88) and the Gulf wars (1991 and 2003). The Iraqi–Iranian war happened while I was a child; therefore I do not have a lot of detailed memories; however, I will try to give a brief account on the life during the Gulf War.

● The war's aftermath

In the years following the 1991 Gulf War, Iraq started to rebuild its damaged infrastructure. Bridges, hospitals and schools were rebuilt. The health services witnessed some improvement after medical supplies were allowed to enter Iraq under the direct supervision of the United Nations; yet, the health services were far behind the rest of the world. Iraq, which is one of the most oil rich countries in the world, was not much better than many of the underdeveloped countries in Africa. There was a big gap between the poor and the rich. The average monthly salary for the vast majority of the people was no more than $5. While people were starving, palaces continued to be built for Saddam's family and supporters. The Ministry of Trade used to provide each person with some essentials like flour, milk and beans (as a source of protein instead of meat). These supplies did not last for more than 2 weeks. Most of the children admitted to hospitals were malnourished and dehydrated. The unjust Iraqi government and the economic sanctions hindered any chance of catching up with nearby countries.

The Iraqi security forces played an important role in maintaining the powerful grip of the Ba'ath Party which ruled the country. There were many punitive military raids against the rebels who fled to the marsh area in the south of Iraq. At that time, not

CASE STUDY

The second Gulf War

In 2003, the second Gulf War started. The war was meant to put an end to Saddam's regime and to target only military bases not the civilians; yet, hospitals over-flowed with civilian causalities. Patients were everywhere. Patients had to share beds due to lack of space. The floor was covered with sheets (not very clean though) and was used as a day surgery to nurse wounded patients. My hospital, Basra Teaching Hospital, which is the biggest hospital in the south of Iraq, ran out of essential medical supplies like syringes, bandages and intravenous fluids. Many died miserably because of blood loss. Surgery had to be done with the aid of kerosene lamps. The war lasted for a few weeks but the country was left in a mess afterwards (see Fig. 11.3). The end of Saddam's regime brought happiness to many suffering Iraqis and it heralded the beginning of a new era in Iraq history.

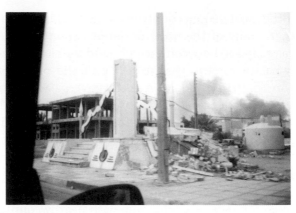

Fig. 11.3 Destruction in the aftermath of war.

being a member of the Ba'ath party was sufficient reason to take a person to execution. Having a relative abroad, for example in the UK, meant a death sentence. One summer day, I witnessed the execution of a row of hand-chained detainees in public. The punishment for not joining the mandatory military service was cutting off ears. There were hundreds of secret jails with thousands of prisoners who suffered all kinds of torture and anguish. The situation moved from bad to worse and many families fled the country to apply for asylum in other countries, although they were chased by the Iraqi security police.

Education deteriorated during that period. Libraries were filled with books, but most of them were old editions. The internet was a big evil according to Saddam's regime as it might open people's minds to what was going on in the rest of the world. Both the United Nations sanctions and the government kept Iraqis isolated and illiterate. No one was allowed to listen to foreign media unless he wanted his wife to be a widow. Bribery even spread to involve the education sector. Teachers could not live on their salary so they had to give private lessons and encouraged students to have them. Many parents forced their children to work rather than attend school. When I came to the UK to do my MSc degree, I discovered how poor we are in

Iraq in teaching techniques. Teaching in Iraq still follows the old style of forcing students to learn rather than making teaching an interactive experience. The lack of security and the unstable situation put off a lot of educated Iraqis who lived abroad from returning back. Many well-known doctors and scientists fled the country.

● The war's aftermath

After the end of Saddam's regime, many families who were living in camps or those who had escaped from Saddam's dictatorship, returned to Iraq. This was added to the ongoing population growth and poor living conditions and further worsened the quality of life in Iraq. Another problem that worsened the health crisis was the extensive administrative corruption. Rebuilding programmes had far less impact than expected. Corruption in Iraq started from petty officials asking for bribes to process a passport all the way up to ministers and high officials. The lack of a central government and the unguarded borders led the country to be a fertile area for terrorism. Car bombs and suicide attacks targeted innocent people. Things are gradually improving. However, it is a very slow process but there are signs of light at the end of the tunnel for Iraqis to resume their lost happiness again.

Summary

Taking Iraq as an example, one can conclude that wars affect nations in many ways. Doctors have to be ready to expect all types of barriers when trying to offer medical expertise in disasters. Wars go beyond mere military actions or civilian death to harm societies in their health services, education, economy, environment and human resources, and the consequences of wars may last for years before normal life returns.

12 The hazards of the job

David Lloyd Roberts

In a short chapter, all we can hope to achieve is to highlight the common features of safety and security that might apply to aid workers when working in conflict areas.

> ⚡ **HAZARD**
>
> It is strongly recommended that you take the time to read up on the threats in more detail from the resources list and take further advice once you arrive in the field.

● Personal security

It is unlikely that you will find yourself in a conflict zone unless you wanted to be there. What I am getting at, is that you volunteered for the work, so you would have given the matter some serious thought. In conflict, there are inherent dangers. You owe it to yourself to know what the dangers are and how to minimize them. When you volunteer, you will see that your contract with whatever organization you are working for mentions at some point that you accept the risks inherent in your work. Before you deploy into a conflict zone any organization worth its salt will ensure that its employees receive security training and detailed briefings on the situation.

What else can you do to help yourself?

● Adjusting

You will need to adjust to your new surroundings as quickly as possible. It's in the first days and weeks of an assignment in a conflict zone that you are at your most vulnerable. Your normal habits and behaviour could now get you into trouble. It's also worth remembering that security mistakes on your part could put any team you are working with in danger. What do we mean?

Take an example from your normal routine: you have had a busy day, you are driving home bumper to bumper as usual, and your radio is playing. On routine occasions like this, your car might be in gear but your mind is pretty much in neutral.

In your new situation, you cannot afford to behave like this. From the moment you arrive at your new destination you should say to yourself, **'Adjust and switch on'.** You must be fully aware of exactly what is happening around you. You must be alert. You must try to think ahead in order to avoid problems and possible danger.

even if you are the passenger, you should take an interest in your immediate surroundings; think about where you might take shelter or find cover if you need it. As you might imagine, this represents a quantum leap from your normal behaviour and lifestyle. If you behaved like this at home, your friends might have some doubts about your sanity! But you are not at home, you are in a conflict zone.

If you make a conscious effort, it is surprising how quickly your natural survival instincts will kick in and how quickly you will be able to adjust. As a result, you will be much safer in your new environment and so will any team you are working with.

● Be inquisitive

In the early days of your mission, make a concerted effort to get as much information as you can about your new environment – the risks, the threats – as it is one of the best ways to improve your security. There will of course be dangers, but if you have a basic understanding of them, they can be avoided or certainly reduced. As the old saying goes, **'Knowledge dispels fear'**. Sometimes newcomers to an organization are a little afraid to be seen as being over-concerned or frightened and so they might hold back from asking for advice or information. This is a mistake; don't be embarrassed to ask questions. Ask your boss, colleagues, the local staff and even the armed forces. With this knowledge comes the confidence you need to get on with your work and to start making a valuable contribution without being a liability to yourself and your fellow team members.

● Forget heroics

You have volunteered to work in a war zone and that's brave enough. Don't get carried away with ideas of changing the world – you won't. You can make a valuable contribution but if you take on too much, if you get too involved in matters that you have absolutely no control over, you will quickly grind yourself into the deck. There will be so much that you feel you have to do. You must prioritize and you must assess the risks involved for almost every event. If you have any doubts about a particular mission or task, don't press on regardless, relying on good luck. Intuition is a valuable gift that we sometimes ignore. If it is telling you something is not as it should be – why not pay attention? You might decide to get more advice from others around you. You might decide to postpone a mission if it appears too risky. It is far more sensible to show moral courage than to press on regardless, thereby possibly putting yourself and others at risk.

Tomorrow is another day. Reassess the risk and if it really seems reasonable, then proceed. Avoid heroics. Being a hero might get you into trouble, which is bad enough, but even worse, it might jeopardize the whole operation. Sometimes it is necessary to protect yourself first in order to be able to protect the victims of conflict later.

Take the time to plan any field mission. Define your aim. What dangers are involved? How far is it, how long will it take? Consider administrative requirements, communications and emergency drills.

PEARL OF WISDOM

Remember the 7 Planning P's:
Prior
Preparation and
Planning
Prevents
Pathetically
Poor
Performance

● Take care of yourself

At some stage of a mission, it is quite likely that you will suffer from the stress of living and working in a conflict environment. You can help yourself by eating properly, getting adequate sleep, avoiding alcohol and making sure you take regular breaks. Don't fall into the trap of thinking you are invincible – you are not and if you don't take care of yourself your performance will rapidly decline. You will become a burden to your colleagues and useless to the people you have come to help.

PEARL OF WISDOM

You are ultimately the guardian of your own security. Knowledge of the threats puts you in a better position to define that important line in the sand, which it is perhaps too dangerous for you, or those in your charge, to cross.

● The conflict environment

The conflict environment in which aid workers have to operate has changed considerably in recent years. The confrontation is now of an 'asymmetric' nature with no clear front lines, with a variety of actors and an impact which is not limited to a given geographical area. Pressures on all actors to choose their sides have increased – 'You are either for us or against us'. In the post 9/11 world there is the perception that humanitarian action has been 'politicized' or some talk of it being 'instrumentalized'. This brings with it the possibility of a dangerous blurring of the lines between core principles of neutral, independent, impartial humanitarian action and military or foreign policy objectives.

● The aid worker as a target

Because of this perception, those who identify aid workers, particularly western aid workers, with the policies of combatants or governments, see them as legitimate targets. Humanitarian action relies very much on the application of international law by all parties to a conflict. In recent years, this law has been abused, misused and, sadly, as a result its credibility has been greatly diminished. The principle that people have a right to humanitarian assistance has come under increasing pressure and the anarchy in certain countries makes them an extremely dangerous working environment for aid workers.

About 10 years ago most aid workers could operate relatively safely in conflict zones as long as they applied some common sense rules. The Red Cross/Crescent as well as other logos used by aid organizations were respected. Now, sadly, quite often they become aiming marks. It is widely held that humanitarian work is becoming more dangerous. There is talk of aid workers being 'soft targets'. In fact, statistics show that the total numbers of security incidents involving aid workers are falling. The significant aspect of the figures, however, is the nature of the incidents. While the number of incidents may be dropping, there is certainly a new and very worrying phenomenon facing the humanitarian worker.

What appears to be happening is that the number of serious incidents involving direct targeting is increasing. So while there might be fewer incidents, overall the nature of these incidents is tending to be more serious. Although this phenomenon is not new, the trend, deliberateness and lethality, has accelerated sharply in recent years. There are a number of reasons for this. There are far more NGOs in existence now than 10 years ago. Therefore, more aid workers are exposed to risk and there are consequently likely to be more incidents. Again, because of the 'global war on terror', the unwritten agreements that allowed aid workers to operate no longer exist in some parts of the world.

'In the past, armed groups might have seen some advantage in the presence of humanitarian actors because of their own interest in protecting and assisting non-combatants in the areas they controlled. In conflicts where mobile and clandestine extremist groups control no territory and do not necessarily aspire to control any... the presence of humanitarians may be perceived as more of a nuisance than an asset.' (Donini, Minera and Walker, 2004, p. 5).

So is the security situation that bad or are aid organizations over-reacting? We need to keep a balance. I have been on missions in most of the recent conflict zones and my honest opinion is that there is a great deal of respect for aid workers. In many countries we are able to carry out our work with the gratitude and support of the local population. There have been tragic incidents in recent years – some a result of poor security practices; others no doubt the result of direct targeting. However, it is important to keep things in proportion. Violent attacks and shooting incidents are commonplace in our cities. Such incidents relating to aid workers are thankfully much rarer. The civilian population understand that the aid provided is often vital to their survival. They need your help and respect you for offering it. As for the military and other armed groups, this respect runs even deeper because they understand the risks you are taking.

THINKING POINT

It is very important to realize that there are certain areas of the world where for the reasons described above it has become almost too dangerous to operate. There is a balance to be struck in such environments between the time and effort spent on remaining secure and what, if anything, can be usefully achieved in terms of humanitarian assistance. Afghanistan, Iraq and certain areas of Sudan spring to mind. Your organization will brief you on such specific areas and the risks involved.

● Other security problems facing aid workers in conflict zones

The blurring of roles between aid workers and the military

Traditionally in conflict situations, there has been a distinction between the military and the non-military domains. Recently, however, military forces have become increasingly involved in traditional humanitarian activities including the provision of aid and medical assistance to the local population. The conflicts in Afghanistan and Iraq, have highlighted certain areas where the military assume a major role in relief assistance.

These developments, coupled with military interventions claimed for humanitarian purposes, have led to an erosion of the separation between the humanitarian and military 'space' and may threaten to blur the fundamental distinction between the two. Aid workers believe this has had a dramatic impact on their security. It has caused a blurring and confusion in their mandate to work in an independent neutral and impartial way for the benefit of the victims. Since armed forces are subordinated to a political mission, they cannot be neutral. However, if aid workers are not perceived as neutral in a conflict, their impartiality and trustworthiness will be in doubt. Their access to people in need, as well as their own security will be put in jeopardy. Associating with a military force in a conflict zone, even by default, implies that the agency in question is in some way identifying with that group, against others. When this association becomes too close, local hostility may result, e.g. The Former Republic of Yugoslavia in the 1990s, Somalia in 1993 and more recently in Afghanistan, Iraq and Darfur.

The hearts and minds issues

Military 'hearts and minds operations', can blur with humanitarian operations. The military aim is to secure the support of certain groups because they live in a certain place and are friendly or potentially so. This strategy might ignore those who are most in need, but who do not constitute a priority for military planners. Within a country, this might easily cause jealousy and resentment between tribes, clans, etc. That could rebound later on NGOs operating in the area. The extensive use of the military in the provision of humanitarian assistance (for example the Provincial Reconstruction Teams [PRTs] in operation in Afghanistan) can make it difficult for opposing parties and the local population to distinguish between independent aid organizations and opposing military forces. This can strip aid workers of their perceived neutrality and they can become targets for the warring factions. Serious problems can arise when these military teams deploy in white four by four vehicles, wearing civilian clothes and carrying weapons. It is hardly surprising if the local people confuse them with aid workers who, apart from the weapons, must look very much the same. Further problems occur when military forces offer aid with 'strings attached', for example in return for intelligence information. The problem therefore is not so much that the military become involved in humanitarian activities, it is when the military link their 'humanitarian operations' to political and military objectives, i.e. when they conduct their activities in a 'camouflaged' way giving the local population the idea that they are aid workers.

Most aid workers accept that on occasions the military must get involved if they are the only ones able to provide assistance, such as when the military are the first to reach a war-affected region or a disaster zone. There are a number of examples of this direct involvement in recent history, e.g. Northern Iraq in April 1991, Kosovo in April 1999 and the Asian tsunami in December 2004. Thus, the blurring issue is many-faceted and has important security implications for aid workers.

Banditry and crime

There will always be those on the fringes of conflict ready to take advantage of the circumstances. Bandits and criminals are unlikely to be under any form of control. They might simply be acting out of self-interest. Emblems used by your organization are unlikely to be respected. Your perceived vulnerability increases the risk and organizations must do what they can to appear a difficult target by the use of protective measures such as physical barriers, alarms, guards, etc.

 HAZARD

We have to treat the threat from bandits and criminals with the greatest caution. **Do not resist if they attempt to rob you.** Also avoid or at least do not prolong a discussion with a drunken soldier. He has a weapon – he will win the argument!

Child soldiers

More and more child soldiers are being used in modern conflicts. Although international humanitarian law prohibits the recruitment of children under the age of 15 into the armed forces, the law is often abused. These children can pose a considerable threat to aid workers particularly when they are trying to impress their superiors and even more particularly when they are fed on a diet of alcohol and drugs. Treat these child soldiers with the utmost caution and, if possible, give them a wide berth.

● The main threats to your security
The mine threat

There are two types of mine: anti-personnel and anti-tank or anti-vehicle mines. The golden rule is that mines and aid workers don't mix. How do we avoid them?

- **Never touch a mine** – stay well clear. Aid workers have been known to move anti-tank mines from a road to gain access. Don't ever try it, they might have built-in anti-handling devices which will explode at the slightest movement. Mines can be attached to trip wires, so again don't take a closer look.

- **Avoid using your radio**, mobile phone or satellite communications equipment (SATCOM) in the proximity of mines (100 m).The radio frequency might cause the mine to detonate.
- **Seek local advice** if moving into a new area or one that has been the scene of recent fighting. Take a guide with you. Ideally, they should be in their own vehicle driving in front, so they are responsible for you.
- **Don't use a track or road that is new to you** unless you are certain others have used it recently. Try not to be the first vehicle to take a road in the morning. Wait and see whether locals are using it, then go. Always wear a seat belt. Avoid driving at night.
- If you are driving and you come across mines, **do not turn your vehicle round**, carefully reverse back along your original path. Do not get out of your vehicle. If the road is blocked, do not be tempted to drive onto the verge as it could contain mines. Similarly, if you meet an oncoming vehicle on a narrow road do not give way by driving onto the verge. Reverse back to a wider area and let the vehicle pass.
- **Try to avoid likely mined areas** such as positions abandoned by the military, deserted houses in battle areas (they could be booby-trapped). Avoid attractive areas in deserted villages or towns, for example, wells, gardens and cultivated areas or undamaged houses where you might be tempted to take shelter.
- Always take it with a 'pinch of salt' if you are told an area is 'cleared of mines'. Roads, main squares etc. might be cleared, but it requires an enormous number of men to completely clear even a small village.

Mines are often marked by the parties to a conflict or indeed by local people. Get to know what markings are used in your area. It might be a red flag placed by the side of the road, a pile of stones perhaps painted red or white or an internationally agreed sign.

The threat from artillery and mortar fire

These weapons are what the military term 'indirect fire weapons'. This means that they require some form of adjustment of the rounds to get them onto a target. Therefore, if you hear artillery or mortar fire in your vicinity it might be the first in a series of rounds that are adjusting onto a target. It's important not to wait for the next round to fall, but to take cover immediately. It is unlikely that you will be the target, but during the adjustment process a shell could land on your vehicle or building by accident. If driving in open country you have two options: if the fire is close to you (50–100 m), the best option is to get out and take cover off the road in a ditch or behind the hardest cover available. If the rounds are landing some distance away, then drive on as quickly as possible to clear the area. If you are in a building and rounds start landing on your town or village, move immediately to your pre-planned shelter area and stay there until the all clear is given. Remember, the next round could, just by accident, land on your building.

The threat from rifle or sniper fire

If you are in a vehicle and you come under fire, drive on at best speed. If you think the firing is coming from your front, you should veer to the left or right up a side street. In the countryside veer off to the side, get out and take cover, putting the vehicle between you and the source of the firing. Reversing or turning round is seldom the best course of action. It slows you down and presents an easier target. Having found cover do not be tempted to look up and see what is going on, or at least not initially. Rather, once you have taken cover, crawl a few meters one way or another to help conceal your exact position. If you are in a building stay there, do not be curious and look out of the window. If you can get to your shelter safely then go there. If not, then find the best protection you can by crawling to the middle of the building or hide under a staircase and put as many walls as possible between you and the sound of the gunfire. The factions might fire warning shots towards aid workers to dissuade them from entering an area or to give them a warning of dangers ahead. If shots are fired over your head or in front of your vehicle in this way it might be wise to take the hint and not press on regardless.

The threat from improvised explosive devices

Improvised explosive devices (IEDs) are 'home-made' weapons. In their simplest form, they can be a stick of dynamite with some nails taped around it for added impact. Devices that are more sophisticated might contain hundreds of kilos of explosive. They can be placed at the side of a road, under a culvert, in a parked car or in a vehicle driven by suicide bombers. Some are even hung from the branches of trees overhanging a road. In recent conflicts, camouflaged IEDs covered with hardened foam and painted to look like boulders have been used. IEDs can be initiated by timing mechanisms, by a command-detonated wire or by radio control.

As with artillery, there is no reason why you should face a direct threat from such devices. They have been put in place with considerable skill and sometimes weeks of pre-reconnaissance to determine patterns of movement, in order to directly target opponents. Why bother wasting valuable manpower and scarce equipment on targeting aid workers? The factions can simply stop your car or force entry into your house or office at any time. Another important characteristic of these weapons worth remembering is that they are often positioned in pairs. The idea is to set one off and then wait before setting off the second. Why? Because their adversaries, including troops, vehicles etc. will naturally gather at the scene to deal with the incident. When sufficient people have gathered, then the second device will be set off.

How can you minimize the threat from these devices? Here are some guidelines:

- If driving, try to **distance yourself from obvious targets** such as security-force vehicles. If you are mixed up with a possible target, a bomber will pay scant regard to your safety. Being in the wrong place at the wrong time could put you in great danger.
- If you happen to be near an explosion, avoid or at least **delay any natural impulse to get closer** to investigate or assist. The best advice is to stop, get out of your vehicle and take cover. The reason is that very often the security forces in the vicinity tend to open fire at 'suspects' immediately after an explosion. Civilians, and that could include you, are often caught in the crossfire.
- **Lie low until the situation has stabilized**. Then, do what you can to help the victims. Apart from crossfire, the other argument in favour of caution is of course the danger of a secondary device.

The threat from unexploded military ordnance (UXO)

In conflict areas, you are bound to come across all types of military ordnance (ammunition) that has been used and failed to work properly, that has been discarded by retreating forces, or just lost by soldiers. UXO ranges from aircraft bombs through artillery shells to grenades and rifle ammunition. All should be treated with extreme caution. Ammunition could be in a very unstable state. The fuse of a shell or bomb might simply require a little nudge from you to complete its task! A grenade lying on the ground might only need to be picked up for its safety pin to fall out and explode.

Unexploded cluster bombs

A particularly nasty feature of modern battlefields is the use of cluster bombs. They scatter smaller 'bomblets' (about the size an individual can of tonic) over vast areas of the battlefield and, because of their very high failure rate, many do not explode. They lie on the ground or hang from trees becoming de facto anti-personnel mines, which can explode at the slightest touch.

As with all UXO, the message is clear:

- They are easily recognizable so there is absolutely no excuse for interfering with them.
- Don't be inquisitive, just leave them alone.
- Never be tempted to take them home as souvenirs.
- Report and warn others of any you see.

● Additional aids to your security

- **Cameras** – best not taken with you on field missions. They could get you into trouble with accusations of spying or intelligence gathering.
- **Mobile phones** – don't rely on them for communications. The local network may break down or become overloaded in a conflict situation. Mobile phones only give you one-to-one communication, i.e. others in your team will not be in the picture as to what is being said. Make sure you have alternative radio communications that you can use in an emergency. Beware of phones with camera and video facilities (see the point on cameras above).
- **Do not allow any weapons in your vehicles or offices** – it could associate you with parties to the conflict and put you in danger.

At check points/road blocks:

- Lower the volume on your radio and obey any signs or instructions to slow down.
- Be polite, friendly and confident. Don't be in a rush to press on.
- Avoid temptation by ensuring all attractive items are out of sight.

● Incident reporting

Incidents may occur in your area and you may be directly involved. So how should you react? Many organizations have their own detailed formats for incident reporting and if they do then of course you should use them. If they do not, then you might use the following guidelines.

The basic idea is to get the required information, quickly and efficiently passed to those who need it or might be in a position to offer immediate help. Again, it's a matter of discipline, the situation might be tense and it is easy to forget important details. A simple format will help you to remember what to report in these trying situations.

It saves valuable time. Because you cover all-important aspects, there is no need for follow-up queries and questions. This can save lives. You should inform your base or colleagues who are in radio contact as soon as possible of the following incident details:

L **LEARNING POINTS**

Incident reporting
WHO – was involved.
WHEN – it happened.
WHERE – it happened.
WHAT HAPPENED – type of incident, any injuries, etc.
FUTURE INTENTIONS – what you now intend doing, do you require assistance?

In a very short and sharp format, you have given all the immediate information you can. Others can now react and you can get on with the problem without the interminable follow-up radio chatter, which just wastes time.

Summary

- When you volunteer for work in a conflict zone, be prepared to:
  - quickly adjust to your new surroundings
  - be inquisitive and get as much information on the security situation as you can
  - avoid heroics but show moral courage
  - take care of yourself.
- In certain countries, western aid workers are perceived as tools of their governments and as such are regarded as legitimate targets by opposition forces.
- Statistics show that the total number of security incidents involving aid workers is falling. However, the number of serious incidents involving direct targeting is increasing. So while there might be fewer incidents overall, the nature of these incidents is tending to be more serious.
- Whereas serious incidents do occur in certain countries, in the rest of the world aid workers are able to carry out their work very much as before with the respect, support and gratitude of the victims of armed conflict.
- The erosion of the separation between humanitarian and military 'space' may threaten to blur the fundamental distinction between the two. This could affect aid workers' security.
- In any conflict zone the main threats to your security such as mines, remain much the same. By having a basic understanding of how they are used, the dangers they pose can be avoided or at least dramatically reduced.

REFERENCES AND FURTHER READING

Reference
Donini A, Minera L and Walker P. The future of
humanitarian action: mapping the implications of Iraq
and other recent crises. *Disasters* 2004; **28** (2): 190–204.

Further reading
*Staying Alive – Safety and Security Guidelines for
Humanitarian Workers in Conflict Zones*. ICRC
Publications, 2005.

ECHO Security Review 2004 – http:?//europa.eu.int/
comm./echo/index_en.htm

David Lloyd Roberts served as a Delegate to the ICRC
advising on operational humanitarian security issues
between 1992 and 2009. This chapter draws on his
experiences of conflict and summarizes key issues from
his book *Staying Alive* written for the ICRC, which they
have kindly agreed may be adapted for this publication.

The ethics of Disaster Medicine

Daniel K. Sokol

● Introduction

For most of us, most of the time, acting ethically is no arduous task. The ethical issues we encounter in our day-to-day lives are quite ordinary: Should I drop a coin in this homeless person's hat? Shall I tell a host that the dish she has laboriously prepared tastes like feet? Is it ethically permissible to steal paper from work for my home printer? These are real ethical issues, but they do not involve life-or-death decisions. The cost of getting it wrong is not usually catastrophic: a feeling of guilt, a disapproving look, perhaps a telling off.

The nurse's dilemma in the case study above arose from an external human threat: advancing enemy troops. At times, the threat is non-human; a tsunami, a tornado, an earthquake, or at the other extreme of size, a pathogen. When Kikwit General Hospital (Democratic Republic of Congo) admitted patients suffering from Ebola haemorrhagic fever (EHF) in 1995, the staff did not forget the decimation of the 1976 Ebola outbreak in the small town of Yambuku, where 11 of the 17 hospital workers were infected and died. EHF is an acute viral illness with a lethality rate ranging from 50 per cent to 90 per cent. In Kikwit, most of the healthcare workers fled the hospital, leaving their patients behind. When Dr Tom Ksiazek of the Special Pathogens Branch of the Centers for Disease Control and Prevention (USA) arrived at Kikwit General Hospital, he

CASE STUDY

An ethical dilemma

In disasters, clinicians and aid workers may be faced with the most difficult of ethical problems. In June 2002, in a large hospital in Toronto, an elderly patient dying from liver cancer asked to see the clinical ethicist. When the ethicist arrived at her bedside, she recounted an experience from January 1942. She was working as a nurse in a military hospital in Penang, Malaysia. The Japanese Imperial Army were advancing on their position and hospital staff were asked to evacuate the residents. They were to walk 11 miles to be collected by British ships.

Though illness or injury, 126 patients were unable to leave the hospital. They would probably be killed with bayonets by the Japanese soldiers. Aware of their fate, some patients asked the medical staff to give them lethal medication. Others asked for hand grenades so they could fight until the bitter end.

What would you do, as a clinician, in such a situation? Would you euthanize a patient too burnt to commit suicide? Would you provide the hand grenades? Sixty years later, the nurse still struggled with her decision to abandon her patients. By fleeing the hospital with the others, did she fail in her duty of care?

found a facility bereft of clinicians but with patients, still living, sharing beds with corpses. For those doctors and nurses, the duty of care did not extend to such drastic situations.

So wide-ranging is the field of disaster medicine and so varied are the types of disasters that can befall humankind that it would be foolish to attempt to identify, let alone address, all the relevant ethical challenges in a single chapter. As Disaster Medicine is a new discipline, medical ethicists have not yet

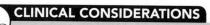

CLINICAL CONSIDERATIONS

The question of the limits of clinicians' duty of care is highly pertinent in the current climate, where severe acute respiratory distress syndrome (SARS), pandemic avian influenza and other emerging diseases are appearing, or expected to appear, in western hospitals. I have elsewhere argued that the duty of care is not limitless, but contingent on a number of factors such as the healthcare worker's speciality (an ophthalmologist may reasonably expect a lower degree of risk than an infectious disease specialist), the risks of harm to the clinician, the likelihood and degree of benefit to the patient if treated and the strength of competing moral obligations associated with other non-clinician roles, such as parent, spouse, carer and so on. A doctor may have a duty to his patients but, as a parent, he may also have duties to his children and in disaster situations these two obligations may conflict.

devoted much attention to the ethical aspects of many disaster situations, save for some work on military medical ethics (Gross, 2006). This, I hope, will change. As mentioned earlier, conflicts and catastrophes present some of the most complex and intractable ethical issues. In this chapter, I present a framework (the **four principles approach**, see below) which may assist healthcare workers in making ethical decisions and provide examples from disaster situations to illustrate the application of the principles and their potential conflict. I conclude with a brief discussion of virtues and their role in Disaster Medicine.

● A framework for ethical decision-making

For centuries, philosophers and theologians have debated the nature of morality. How can we determine that a particular act – stealing an apple from the market stall, for example – is morally right or wrong? Scholars have proposed many answers. One group claims that it is wrong because God (or gods) says it's wrong. Proponents of this view may point to the eighth commandment: thou shalt not steal. For this group, it is divine command that determines the rightness or wrongness of an act. Another group, generally labelled **consequentialists**, believe that the rightness or wrongness of an act depends solely on the consequences. For them, stealing an apple is right if it leads to a better state of affairs overall than not stealing the apple. Hence a father who stole the apple from a rich farmer to feed his starving family may have acted rightly, especially if no one else noticed the theft. Another group (called **deontologists**), while acknowledging the moral importance of consequences, may focus on the fulfilment of certain rights and duties. Most deontologists would claim that stealing an apple is wrong because we have a duty not to steal other people's property, although this prohibition can on occasion be trumped by other duties, such as the duty to prevent great harm to loved ones. The disputes between these families of moral theories continue unabated and sophisticated versions and modifications of each theory still emerge in philosophical journals.

In the late 1970s, two American philosophers, Tom Beauchamp and James Childress, published a textbook introducing an approach to medical ethics which has since dominated the field. In their *Principles of Biomedical Ethics*, now in its sixth edition, they present four principles which they claim are compatible with a range of moral theories and which, collectively, capture the whole of medical morality. In the section below, I describe each of the principles and discuss their relevance to Disaster Medicine.

The principle of respect for autonomy

The word 'autonomy' literally means 'self-rule'. Clinicians have an obligation to respect the deliberated self-rule of moral agents, in particular of patients under their care. More specific rules can be derived from this general principle. Most obviously, clinicians should obtain informed consent before performing procedures or giving medication to patients. When you propose to do something to a competent person, you must give them enough information to make a considered decision and seek their permission. Another obligation is to respect patient confidentiality, since an implicit promise of secrecy exists between patient and clinician. When I visit my general practitioner, I do not expect him to tell his friends about my thrombosed external piles. The principle of respect for autonomy also rules out deception, for patients cannot make proper decisions if presented with an inaccurate picture of the world. They must have true, relevant facts. The principle also requires the clinician to have good communication skills, for there is little point in providing information if it is not understood by the patient.

In a disaster situation, these requirements may be hard to fulfil. Obtaining informed consent requires time, but spending time to obtain permission from one patient may endanger the health of others. Respecting confidentiality or privacy may be impossible or unrealistic in battlefield situations or in crowded refugee camps. If posted abroad, the clinician may not speak the patient's language or dialect and no interpreter may be available. In the face of a dreadful situation, it may be cruel to share depressing news and extinguish hope: for example, that no help is coming or that death from traumatic injury awaits. Truth-telling may be inhumane in some circumstances. James Orbinski, a physician working with Médecins Sans Frontières during the Rwandan genocide, recalls what he saw outside a hospital in June 1994:

> People all around us writhed and screamed in pain. Others lay dead as relatives and friends wailed. There were hundred of casualties. There were people with gunshot wounds, machete blows, shrapnel and blast injuries. There were women and girls who had been raped. The wounded came in wave after wave (Orbinski, 2008, pp. 225–6).

In such situations, the principle of respecting individual autonomy is of secondary importance. The principle of justice (see below) requires you to allocate your time and resources to benefit as many of the wounded as possible. You would be morally justified, if faced with a patient's autonomous request for time-consuming treatment, to decline in favour of treating others. The same is true if, following the detonation of a suicide bomb in a bus, several polytrauma patients arrived through your hospital doors, each requiring urgent surgical intervention. Invoking the 'life before limb' maxim, you may justifiably refuse to save the leg of a patient whose life is not in immediate danger in order to save the life of another patient, however much that first patient may protest.

Respect for autonomy usually refers to the autonomy of patients, but it may apply to others' autonomy too. Military doctors, for example, may face potentially conflicting obligations to respect the orders of their commanders and respect the autonomy of their patients. A 2003 US military memorandum on the use of aggressive interrogation techniques stressed that the detainee must be 'medically evaluated as suitable' and that 'qualified medical personnel' must be present during interrogations. The situation described earlier when healthcare staff abandon their workplace during virulent epidemics represents another conflict between respecting the autonomy of patients (who may well wish to be treated) and clinicians' autonomous desire to protect themselves and loved ones from risk of harm.

The fact that the requirements of respect for autonomy can conflict (e.g. respecting the autonomy of one patient may entail violating the autonomy of another) reveals that the obligation to respect autonomy is not absolute, but *prima facie*. In other words, the duty is binding unless it conflicts with a weightier moral duty. Hence, in the case of torture, a physician may justifiably violate the autonomous instruction of his superior if he believes such an order represents a breach of humanitarian and public international law (legal justice), international codes of medical ethics (notably the World Medical Association's Declaration of Tokyo), fundamental human rights (rights-based justice) and the principles of beneficence and non-maleficence. We turn now to these two principles.

The principles of beneficence and non-maleficence

 THINKING POINT

Many readers will be familiar with the Hippocratic Oath, the ancient Greek text written nearly 2500 years ago. One section describes the duties of a doctor: 'I will use treatments for the benefit of the ill in accordance with my ability and my judgment but from what is to their harm or injustice I will keep them.'

While the Hippocratic Oath may not sound contentious, doctors have on many occasions violated these tenets. Healthcare professionals have and still do, participate in torture and executions, often justifying their participation by claiming that they are preventing harm to others or promoting a greater good. Thus American medical personnel did not administer painkillers during the interrogation of Al Qaeda leader Abu Zubaydah, even though he had been shot in the groin during his capture. Only once the interrogation was over did they relieve his pain (Gross, 2006, p. 232). This is a gross violation of the spirit of medicine, so clearly exposed in the extract from the Oath.

The spirit of benevolence is captured in the actions of the Chechen surgeon Hasan Baiyev who, finding the Chechen warlord Shamil Basayev severely wounded from a mine, applied local anaesthetic and amputated his right leg. The operation done, the rebels took their leader into the Caucasian mountains. Threatened by Russians troops who complained that he had helped the patient flee, Dr Baiyev noted that he had followed the Hippocratic Oath, helping Russians and Chechens alike.

The principle of beneficence requires clinicians to act in the best interests of their patients. Non-maleficence states that they should refrain from causing them net harm – *net* harm because most interventions and indeed most attempts to help others, run the risk of harm. Surgery, with its obligatory incision or drilling, would otherwise defy the principle of non-maleficence. In the context of healthcare, both principles are usually considered together, translated into a commitment to benefit patients with minimum harm.

Clinicians respectful of these two principles will, amongst other qualities, be competent (they must be able to perform the procedures in a manner that will help rather than harm), will exercise sound judgement (for example, to determine whether a risky operation is needed in the circumstances), will recognize the limits of their competence – including realizing when 'having a go' at operations beyond their expertise, though tempting, is ill-advised and knowing when to refer to more suitable experts – (see Chapter 8), will respect patient autonomy (because people's conception of benefit is to some extent particular to the individual), will attend courses for their continuous professional development (such as, in the UK, the Diploma in Tropical Medicine of the London School of Hygiene and Tropical Medicine, or the Diploma in the Medical Care of Catastrophes at the Society of Apothecaries, to ensure patients are provided with up-to-date and effective care), will act responsibly in their privates lives when it may impact their clinical work (e.g. avoiding excessive consumption of alcohol the evening before a delicate operation or engaging in relationships which could disrupt teamwork or the doctor–patient relationship) and will communicate effectively (poor communication can lead to physical and emotional distress).

Even under normal circumstances in wealthy countries, it is not possible to benefit all sick people. Some sick people do not want to be helped and here the principle of respect for patient autonomy (at least in the western context) usually requires us to respect this wish as long as the patient is informed and competent. Even when patients want to be helped, limitations in our medical knowledge may prevent us from curing certain conditions, such as types of cancer and psychiatric disorders. Life-prolonging but expensive medications may not be freely available due to financial constraints, and operations may need to be delayed (with subsequent harm) because we do not have enough operating theatres or specialist surgeons. The resource constraints are usually exacerbated in times of disaster, resulting in troubling decisions about who to prioritize.

HAZARD

In developing countries, when resources do become available, perhaps as a result of a sudden influx of international aid following a disaster, the local population may benefit from interventions not normally available. However, when the initial crisis subsides and the media's attention is diverted elsewhere, the aid tends to evaporate and appropriate follow-up may not be available. The degree of benefit is curtailed by a premature exit. Some orthopaedic patients from the earthquake that struck Pakistan and killed around 80000 people in October 2005 are still wearing external fixators.

To confer greater benefit to patients and avoid accusations of abandonment, medical aid organizations should ideally plan beyond the immediate into the longer term, although the unpredictability of disasters, the situation on the ground and various logistical considerations may make such planning difficult.

Many governments, anticipating the arrival of pandemic influenza, are pondering ways to resolve the moral dilemmas that will emerge when the health service is stretched beyond capacity. Who should get vaccinated first? Who should get the few intensive care beds and ventilators? Should healthcare workers and key figures in society get priority? Which medical services should be closed down first? How can we avoid social unrest? The principles of beneficence and non-maleficence may require selecting options likely to lead to the most good and the least harm overall, thus prioritizing patients who have the best chance of recovery, who may contribute to the collective effort (such as doctors, nurses, paramedics and so on) or who may be essential to the proper functioning of the country. The question then is: is this a fair way to choose who lives and who dies? In other words, what criteria of justice should we use to make these decisions? More on this follows below.

The principle of beneficence should also encourage clinicians to try to get others, be they governments, pharmaceutical companies, or individuals, to see the full horror and injustice of a situation and to act on this awareness to improve conditions on the ground. In Malawi, for example, AIDS is so prevalent that the average life expectancy is 36 years (Orbinski, 2008).

The principle of beneficence may also require clinicians to share their stories and lessons learnt from their experiences in journals, books, lectures and other fora to help others deal more effectively with similar conflicts and catastrophes in the future. Cancio and Pruitt, for example, by examining published

THINKING POINT

We should strive to persuade pharmaceutical companies to develop more drugs for diseases affecting the developing world, to license some of their patents to local producers who can develop drugs at a fraction of the price and to reduce their profit margins if this means more affordable drugs and the prevention of thousands of premature deaths. For clinicians, treating patients in the old fashioned way, one by one, is not the only means of benefiting the sick.

accounts of recent mass casualty burn disasters, have derived a set of principles for the management of future burn incidents, including lessons on disaster planning, control and communication, triage, transport, treatment, personnel management, supplies and rehabilitation (Cancio and Pruitt, 2004). Many valuable lessons have also been learnt from the recent epidemics of SARS and our experiences with Ebola epidemics in Africa have reminded us of the importance of understanding local customs, cultures and traditional healing practices. Learning from colleagues in our own and other disciplines and sharing lessons for the benefit of others are both ethical obligations. The principle of justice, to which we now turn, also calls for the sharing of information, for just as we have benefited from the findings and expertise of others, so too should we contribute to the pool of knowledge.

The principle of justice

This principle requires moral agents to act fairly. There are different types of justice, including *distributive* justice (giving people their fair share of resources), *rights-based* justice (respecting people's human rights) and *legal* justice (respecting the laws of the country). Although we might be tempted to interpret justice as treating people equally, a moment's thought shows this account is lacking. It is possible to treat individuals equally but unjustly, such as by decimating an entire group of people, such as Jews or Tutsis, indiscriminately. It would also be unethical, in some circumstances, to divide scarce medical resources (e.g. our entire stock of antibiotics) equally among the population, since some individuals – those with bacterial infections – are in much greater need of antibiotics than others, most of whom are healthy. In an accident and emergency ward, then, we tend to treat people using a 'first come, first served' rule, but this rule can be overridden. If a patient arrives with blunt trauma to the head he will be treated before a patient with a laceration on his arm, even if the latter was admitted first. Despite losing his turn, this patient is unlikely to complain. He will recognize that the criterion used to justify the unequal treatment is fair; it is one based on medical need.

CASE STUDY

One surgeon for 300 wounded

The problem in a disaster situation is that it may not be possible to satisfy the medical needs of all our patients. The Chechen surgeon, Dr Baiyev, was called to treat 300 soldiers wounded from the fighting between Chechen and Russian troops. As the only surgeon in the town, he conducted over 100 operations in 24 hours, including seven skull surgeries and 67 amputations. He eventually ran out of medication. In this situation, lack of personnel and equipment limited the ability to meet medical need. In war time, however, medical need may be trumped by a broader objective.

In some limited military contexts, medical need is secondary to the need to return troops to duty. Intensive medical efforts on wounded soldiers who have no prospects of a return to the front, when such efforts could be directed at less seriously injured soldiers, weakens the fighting force and risks undermining the war effort. Military need, or the common good, can take precedence over individual medical need.

Even in civilian settings, the medical needs of an individual can be overridden during mass-casualty incidents (MCI). When many people are severely injured and saving the one patient with the greatest medical need entails the death of several others with lesser need, it may be justifiable to apply the consequentialist maxim 'the greatest good for the greatest number'. The P4 Expectant category (i.e. expected to die) used in triage during MCIs does not necessarily mean that the patient could not be saved in 'normal' circumstances. Hirshberg, Holcomb and Mattox observe:

> A critically injured patient may be directed into a shock room if he or she is one of the first casualties to arrive at the hospital, whereas a similar patient arriving later will correctly be triaged into the expectant category (Hirshberg, Holcomb and Mattox, 2001, p. 649).

Categorizing the patient as 'expectant' may depend on the resources available at the time (see Chapter 2).

In such situations, the criterion of justice shifts from one based on medical need to one based on welfare-maximization. This shift is also anticipated in the context of pandemic flu, where some medical services will be closed at certain trigger points to focus energies on dealing with the pandemic. The result is that many patients awaiting non-flu-related treatments will not be benefited.

It is not only individuals who are bound by the four principles. **Governments and institutions also have moral responsibilities in disaster planning and response**. Most obviously, they have a duty to plan for disaster situations by considering a range of issues, financial, logistical, organizational and educational. This must include suitable training for relevant medical personnel and, during epidemics, the provision of necessary equipment, such as personal protective equipment (PPE), in order to reduce risks of infection to self and others. It is also important that any measures proposed are perceived to be just by the stakeholders (thus transparency in decision-making is usually desirable), for feelings of injustice can lead to social unrest. During the SARS epidemics in Toronto, some staff were offered 'risk pay' for their high risk exposure. This created resentment and anger from nurses in institutions whose pay was not increased, despite identical risks. This sense of injustice can lead healthcare staff to feel undervalued and may encourage absenteeism, with consequent harms to patients and overworked colleagues.

Using the four principles as a basic moral framework, I have provided an overview of some of the ethical issues that may arise in disaster situations. There are many more to be identified and examined. Although disasters take many different forms, this principle-based approach (sometimes called **principlism**) helps identify key ethical issues and conflicts both within and between the principles. The astute reader will have noted, perhaps with some frustration, that they do not provide an answer. They are not a panacea. Each principle is not absolute, and can be overridden by other principles depending on the context. When principles clash (and they often will during conflicts and catastrophes), the decision-maker will have to use sound judgement to determine which of the moral duties is most compelling in the circumstances. At best, the principles provide an analytic framework which allows us to approach chaotic situations in a rational and systematic manner.

The integrity of the moral decision-making process is essential: you must be able to explain *why* you have come to the conclusion that letting these patients die (seemingly violating the principle of non-maleficence) is justifiable. Perhaps they asked to die, as did some of the doomed patients of the military nurse in Malaysia and you respected their autonomy, or perhaps treating them would result in the preventable death of many others with a stronger claim to your services (justice and beneficence to others), or perhaps treating them would actually worsen their condition and palliation is medically indicated (non-maleficence). Finally, you may leave them to die because, like the clinicians faced with the Ebola virus at Kikwit General Hospital, you feel your duty of self-preservation outweighs your duty of care. This is where distinguishing between *obligatory* and *supererogatory* acts is helpful.

An obligatory act is one that you are morally required to do. If your patient needs antibiotics for his pneumonia, you have, under normal circumstances, an obligation to treat him. A supererogatory act, however, is not obligatory; it goes beyond the call of duty.

CASE STUDY

A supererogatory act

In February 2008, in Helmand Province, Afghanistan, Lance Corporal Matthew Croucher was part of a four-man team exploring a suspected Improvised Explosive Device (IED) factory. Once in the compound, in poor visibility, his leg hit a trip-wire. A grenade fell next to him. Croucher shouted 'Grenade' to warn his companions and threw himself on top of the grenade, placing his rucksack between his body and the grenade. All four men survived. Croucher was awarded a George Cross for his bravery. Croucher's selfless act was supererogatory.

In some disaster situations, the boundaries between the two categories can be fuzzy. It is not always clear when an act ceases to be morally obligatory and encroaches into the supererogatory. Is caring for Ebola patients in an under-resourced hospital with high risk of personal harm and minimal chance of improving prognosis obligatory or beyond the call of duty?

More generally, if doctors are committed to the principles of beneficence and justice, should those working in western countries spend some time in poorer countries where doctors are as rare as unicorns and their services are desperately needed? In 2005, eleven nations in Africa did not have a single neurologist. Is such a benevolent migration from England to Africa, which might well entail foregoing many everyday comforts, obligatory or supererogatory?

> **PEARL OF WISDOM**
>
> 'The only thing necessary for the triumph of evil is for good men to do nothing.' Attributed to Edmund Burke (1729–97).

Individuals who regularly go beyond the call of duty are often described as virtuous. Lance Corporal Croucher, according to senior military officers, displayed outstanding bravery, self-sacrifice, quickness of thought, devotion to duty, and exemplary behaviour. One approach to ethics is centred around the notion of virtues or of the virtuous person. A brief exposition follows.

● Virtue ethics

A virtue ethics approach, unlike principlism, does not focus on the right thing to do, but on moral character. Virtues are traits of character, such as courage, compassion and wisdom, that promote human flourishing. For Aristotle, a founding father of virtue theory, a virtue is the 'golden mean' between two undesirable extremes. At one end of the continuum, you have a vice of excess. At the other, a vice of deficiency. The virtue of courage, for example, lies on the golden mean between the vices of recklessness (excess) and cowardice (deficiency). A virtue ethics approach might ask, 'What kind of person should I be?' or, in a given situation, 'How would a virtuous clinician behave here?' This virtue approach can enrich principlism. Moral action requires a combination of virtues and principles, since a doctor must exercise the virtues of discernment, integrity, benevolence, trustworthiness (and so on) to discharge the duties required by the principles.

CASE STUDY

A combination of virtues and principles

Certain virtues, in particular courage and judgement, are particularly relevant during disasters, when various threats and pressures may lead to cowardice or rash decisions. Dr Matthew Lukwiya, a Ugandan doctor who coordinated the response of St Mary's Hospital during the 2000 Ebola outbreak in Uganda, kept his composure when others were panicking. He informed the health authorities early in the outbreak and set up an isolation ward. His rigid adherence to the guidelines of the World Health Organization helped contain the disease. One day in November, following the deaths of three healthcare workers, 400 staff assembled in protest, some calling for the hospital to close. In an inspirational speech, Dr Lukwiya told his staff that he could not force them to stay, but that he would remain in the hospital, alone if necessary, until the end of the epidemic or the end of his life. The staff stayed. While caring for a sick nurse, Dr Lukwiya contracted Ebola and died on December 5, 2000.

In situations requiring immediate action, such as when a live grenade drops to your feet, there is no time for a detailed analysis of moral principles. You act as you think a good soldier/doctor/nurse/civilian would act. Those training clinicians in disaster medicine, anticipating that trainees may face moral decisions requiring instant action, should find ways to instil these desirable traits of character in trainees, perhaps by studying the virtuous behaviour of others in a range of demanding situations.

When principles yield little comfort or clarity, it is sometimes helpful to ask what a virtuous person, perhaps an inspiring mentor, would do in our shoes. While the virtuous course of action is often obvious, it may not be clear in moral dilemmas and, once again, the decision-maker will be left to make a reasoned judgement.

Summary

Disasters, by their very nature, disturb the normal course of events. Earthquakes, wars, epidemics, or genocides, all catastrophes can threaten human life and welfare in violent ways. In the turmoil, amidst the blood and tears of victims and relatives, lie ethical choices, some so profound that they can affect our very core, the way we perceive ourselves and others. In his haunting account of the Rwandan genocide, in which a million people were killed, James Orbinski writes:

> I lost my questions and for 18 months afterwards existed in a kind of netherworld of confusion, trying to sidestep memories that could impose themselves at any time. I struggled against what I knew and could not escape. I struggled to find a way to understand and regain my footing as a man, as a doctor and as a putative humanitarian. And I still struggle now when I confront memories of that time, memories that are no longer unspeakable, but still unbearable (Orbinski, 2008, p. 163).

However distressing, hard moral choices must not be ignored or dismissed, for only by confronting them can we seek to improve our decision-making when faced with similar choices in the future. As this chapter has shown, we also need to recognize and accept that, at times, every available option will fail to assuage the suffering of all.

In such tragic choices, when even the best option will transgress some moral value, despair and regret are inescapable.

Over a hundred years ago, the philosopher George Santayana noted that 'those who cannot remember the past are condemned to repeat it'. Medicine, from psychiatry to trauma surgery, has learnt much from past disasters. The relatively new field of Medical Ethics can also learn from the extraordinary moral dilemmas encountered by clinicians at the front line. While disasters and suffering will continue until the extinction of our species, I hope ethicists, clinicians and other disaster specialists will work together, sharing ideas, experiences and expertise, to coordinate responses that, while medically and logistically effective, uphold the values of our ever-bruised but noble humanity.

REFERENCES

Cancio L and Pruitt B. Management of mass casualty burn disasters. *International Journal of Disaster Medicine* 2004; **2:** 114–29.

Gross M. *Bioethics and Armed Conflict.* MIT Press, London, 2006.

Hirshberg A, Holcomb J and Mattox K. Hospital trauma care in multiple-casualty incidents: a critical view. *Annals of Emergency Medicine* 2001; **37** (6): 647–52.

Orbinski J. *An Imperfect Offering.* Random House, Toronto, 2008.

14 Electives in the developing world

Mark Wilson

LEARNING POINTS

Basics of elective planning: factors to consider:

- Finding out about places including internet resources
- Funding
- Visas
- Occupational health and immunizations
- Things to take
- Making a career of it
- Useful resources and Further reading

● Introduction

Your elective can be the most rewarding and memorable part of your entire medical training. Spending time once qualified gaining further experience overseas can also be incredibly fulfilling. Planning for such adventures, however, can take many months so early preparation is essential (Fig. 14.1). With today's job application processes being so dependent on 'describing an experience in which you...' type questions, the experiences you gain from your elective may well enable you to give interesting and different answers. There are many things to consider.

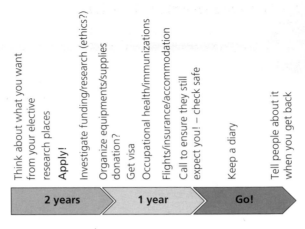

Think about what you want
from your elective

research places

Apply!

Investigate funding/research (ethics?)

Organize equipments/supplies
donation?

Get visa

Occupational health/immunizations

Flights/insurance/accommodation

Call to ensure they still
expect you! – check safe

Keep a diary

Tell people about it
when you get back

| 2 years | 1 year | Go! |

Fig. 14.1 Preparation timeline.

● The basics of elective planning

You can do virtually anything you want for your elective. Even if your University does place restrictions, these can often be overcome if you can justify why you **must** do a specific project. This vast opportunity can make it extremely difficult to know what to do and many students don't know where to start. The important thing though is to think about it early. If in doubt, work through the questions below and then get writing!

● General considerations

THINKING POINT

If the idea of going somewhere without a hairdryer, a local supermarket or Starbucks™ is too much to bear, then you probably need to buy another book! If, however, you relish the chance to get involved with a community with challenges very different to your own, then read on…

Why? – Beware medical tourism

It is worth thinking at the outset about what you want to get out of your period overseas. Do you want to go to a developing country to practise skills that you would not be allowed to do back home? Hang on! Is that right? It's worth spending a few minutes getting this straight in your head. **Medical tourism** in this context refers to the dubious ethical aspects of doing an elective or period of work to 'practise' procedures or medicine. There is no doubt that this is wrong if you are not competent to perform them in your own country. It does not mean that going on an elective is wrong, so long as this is clear in your mind.

The experiences that you should be aiming to gain are those of better understanding of healthcare in a different culture/system with different resources from your own. You will no doubt also experience and gain a greater understanding of a different spectrum of diseases. If competent (or if taught while there) to do various procedures (e.g. chest drains in a trauma setting), you may also perform these and gain technical experience. All this relates to **your experience** – you must also consider **your impact.** In the vast majority of circumstances, your impact will be a very positive one, giving permanent staff a bit of a break while you help out. However, it can be negative – you will consume resources. See the references in the appendix if you want to read around this subject a bit more, but enough of that! Your elective is going to be fun! Just keep it in the back of your mind and don't rack yourself with guilt (save that for the environmental impact of your trip later in this chapter).

When?

For most students, the period to do their elective is set in stone. However, at some universities it is variable. You are more likely to be using your skills independently during your elective than during any other part of your training. For this reason, it is usually best to do your elective as late in your training (when you have the most experience) as possible.

Where?

This is a huge question and involves personal desires, language, safety, affordability, the weather. If you have an interest in a specific condition, have a look at the country profile pages and the global atlas on the World Health Organization's website (www.who.int/globalatlas). These give a very good guide to current disease rates around the world.

THINKING POINTS

- Are you happy to rough it a bit?
- Why am I going? (desire to help/adventure/ experience?)
- Do you speak any other languages?
- Are you (and is your school) okay with you going to areas with high prevalence of trauma/HIV?
- Are you wanting to go alone or with friends?
- Do you want to go to a Mission Hospital?
- Do you also want a holiday?
- Climate
- Cost
- Length of trip
- I'm really serious and want to make Disaster Medicine and developing world work my career (see end of chapter)

Language

Attempting to do psychiatry in remote Mongolia could leave you a little lost unless you are fluent in Mongolian (although you may appear to be a very effective listener!). **FIND OUT** in advance how things work if you don't speak the local language. Many doctors around the world speak English since so many books are written in it; however, you will not be much help if you have to rely on them to translate. In many mission hospitals the nurses double as translators. As a general guide, nurses in East or Southern Africa and India and Pakistan can double as translators. If you're thinking of going to South America or West Africa, you may need to be pretty fluent in Spanish/Portuguese or French respectively. If you're planning far enough in advance, could you attempt to learn at least the basics of the language? The more you put in...

THINKING POINT

In the UK there is one doctor per 629 people. In Mozambique it is 1: 143 350.

Exposure to risk

We are continually exposed to risks. It's normal. At home you balance these risks (not walking through the park at night, wearing a cycle helmet, double-gloving) unconsciously. When you are in a new environment, these risks may not be so apparent and hence require more thought.

HAZARD

Two 'risks' in particular seem to get some medical schools a bit twitched. After all, they have a responsibility for your welfare during their course. The first is **trauma**, and the second is **HIV**.

Understandably, most medical schools are not keen on their students going to countries where there is active conflict. There are countries, however, with a great deal of violence that remain out of the news. Do all you can to find out the current situation if considering going to such a place (visit www.fco.gov.uk for the latest Foreign Office advice). Once there, do all you can to reduce exposure to such risk. It is all too tempting to think that, for example, you don't need a cycle helmet when using a moped in a foreign country! They work just as well! Just because no one else does, it doesn't make it safer for you not to bother!

The second risk many people are concerned about is HIV. Although you may not intend to do any exposure-prone procedures, this may prove impossible if you are repeatedly asked to. If you are going to a place of high HIV prevalence, assume you will be doing at least some procedures. If this makes you feel nervous (maybe because you haven't done much suturing or blood-taking) think hard before going. Certainly consider taking post-exposure prophylaxis (see below) with you.

CLINICAL CONSIDERATIONS

Always use **Universal Precautions** (even if you are a bit lax at home) – this includes wearing goggles and an apron as well as double-gloving – but also maintain a sense of perspective. Accidental needlestick transmission of HIV is very low (approx 0.3 per cent, but is higher for Hep B and C). Don't let fear paralyse you.

● Conflict and catastrophe medicine and non-governmental organizations

Getting involved on the ground with Disaster Medicine as a student can be somewhat difficult. It is important to understand why and not to feel dejected following your offer of 'free' help. First, by definition, the area you aim to go to is resource-poor. Despite your best intentions you will consume resources (water, food, shelter, energy). In addition, at least while you are a student, someone or an organization will have to be responsible for your safety and, when that's following a natural disaster or conflict, it can be very costly. You could also be a target yourself and put others in danger. The amount of training you would require to function and be of benefit in such environments is usually outweighed by the shortness of an elective. For all these reasons, many non-governmental organizations (NGOs) that work in disaster relief do not take medical students on elective. The big players (such as the Red Cross/Crescent [the world's largest humanitarian organization] and Médecins sans Frontières) require minimum work periods of at least 6 months (often a year), usually require the Diploma in Tropical Medicine and Hygiene and often stipulate that volunteers need to be at Registrar level or above.

PEARL OF WISDOM

Some NGOs

Some may not be that receptive to elective students, but there's no harm in talking to them:

- The Red Cross/Crescent www.redcross.int
- African Medical and Research Foundation (AMREF) www.amref.org
- British Nepal Medical trust www.britainnepalmedicaltrust.org.uk
- Médecins sans Frontières www.msf.org
- Raleigh International www.raleighinternational.org

That does not mean you can't be involved at all. First, there are some NGOs that are very glad to take medical students. They are usually small local units providing care from relative safety on the edge of a conflict zone where the conflict has been longstanding (e.g. Thai/Burmese border). Organizing an elective with such a group requires either local contacts or fairly intense research.

● To go it alone or with friends?

The best way to immerse yourself in a new environment is to do so alone, however, this can be daunting and so you may well want to go with someone. It can also make journeys cheaper and safer. This decision will depend on what you want and also if you have any friends!

● Mission/faith hospitals

For many years, missionary hospitals have played a vital role in providing healthcare in remote and resource-poor parts of the world. They have also been common elective destinations. As a rough rule, compared with government-run hospitals, they are often more friendly, especially towards students, and contain like-minded people. If not religious yourself, you may think a mission hospital would be inappropriate for you. They vary greatly in terms of what they expect. Some would ask for nothing more than your respect for those who practise the faith in the hospital; others might expect you to take a more active role. Speak to people who have been there before, look at their website...try to get a feel for the place.

● Other considerations

You should also consider the weather at the time of year you intend to go (for example, if working in the Himalayan foothills of India or Nepal, you could get very cold over winter). Although the cost of flights may deter you from going to a specific place, there are many grants (see below) which should be able to help. And finally, you probably deserve a bit of a break! Think about places you would like to visit en route or on the way back.

● Finding out about places

It is now easier than ever to find hospitals or other institutions. The internet has reduced what used to take three months (searching through elective reports, writing, awaiting a response) to a process that can take an hour – search on the net and send an e-mail. However, the more you put into finding the right place for you, the more you will get out and there is nothing quite like a personal recommendation of a place.

Elective reports/evenings

Most schools keep a bank of elective reports, either online or in the library. Spend an afternoon flicking through these. At your electives evening, people from the year above may be able to tell you about places they have been. They can often give you the best advice.

Senior colleagues

Often Consultants or other seniors will have worked overseas, usually in their area of interest. If you want to listen to lots of heart murmurs from rheumatic fever, ask your cardiologist if he can recommend anywhere. If it's tropical diseases you're after, talk to your microbiologist/infectious disease colleagues. Their recommendation can also serve as a good introduction when you write to the hospital.

Medline, PubMed, Google Scholar

These are great resources if you have a specific area of interest. If you are really interested in doing a malaria project and want to go to Africa – do the search. You will quickly find who is actively doing what you want to be involved in.

The Internet

A Google search will bring up most of what you want. HospitalWeb (http://neuro-www.mgh.harvard.edu/hospitalweb.shtml) provides lists of virtually all hospitals that have a website. MedicsTravel (www.medicstravel.org) lists more and especially those that are more remote without websites. There are websites that are good for specific areas.

Non-Governmental organizations

An NGO is a legally-constituted organization (usually not for profit) created by private persons or organizations with no participation or representation of any government. There are thought to be between one and two million in India alone, hence a comprehensive list is not possible! The World Health Organization (www.who.org) has links to many sites (medical and non-medical). RedR (formerly the International Health Exchange) also has links as well as some very good courses that are worth taking before working for an NGO. A fairly comprehensive list of medical-related NGOs with UK links is kept on: www.medicstravel.org

Missionary and faith organizations

There are some excellent websites listing missionary hospitals. There are also a number of missionary organizations that are more 'student-welcoming' than some of the bigger NGOs:

 LEARNING POINTS

Some Missionary Organizations

- Mission Finder www.mfinder.org
  Two very useful subsections are:
  - For electives: www.missionfinder.org/medstudents.htm
  - For short-term medical work: www.missionfinder.org/medical.htm
- Oscar www.oscar.org.uk
- Health Serve www.healthserve.org (a ministry of the Christian Medical Fellowship www.cmf.org.uk/)
  - The CMF provide a number of extremely good elective guides for doctors, nurses and dentists. They are all available from: http://www.healthserve.org/electives/
- Africa Inland Mission www.aimint.org
- Baptist Missionary Society www.bms.org.uk
- Catholic Medical Missions Board www.cmmb.org
- Christians Abroad www.cabroad.org.uk
- Emmanuel Healthcare (formerly Edinburgh Medical Missionary Society) www.emms.org

- International Nepal Fellowship www.inf.org
- Leprosy Mission www.leprosymission.org

● Applying for an elective

The digital age has meant that it is often cheaper (and certainly quicker) for dialogue between you and your prospective destination to be done electronically than via post. That's not always possible and, if using mail, you should allow a good couple of months to get a reply especially from the more remote areas. Whichever form of communication you use, make sure you write clearly, explain why you are applying to this destination specifically and enclose or attach a CV. Many places will ask for a reference or letter of good standing from your Dean. Some hospitals, especially the ones linked to large medical schools may have an online application process – check before writing.

Over the last 10 years, some medical schools have realized there is money to be made out of electives. This principally started in the US with medical schools such as Harvard charging $3000 per month. Not surprisingly, resource-poor medical schools in Africa and Asia have now also started charging. This is a bit bizarre because (for example in South Africa) they will charge you to go to a rural hospital that they are affiliated with even though they will have nothing to do with your elective. Your own medical school may have had affiliations with that hospital going back many years. If at all possible, try to make sure money you pay or a donation that you want to give goes directly to the place you are working at.

● Grants and funding

There are literally hundreds of grants available for medical students. Many of these do not actually get awarded due to lack of applications every year. There are lists on a number of websites, but the BMA website (www.bma.org.uk/ap.nsf/ Content/Medicalelectivescontactinfo) is a good place to start. There are also many other grants that are not specific for electives: www.rdinfo.org.uk is an excellent source for these.

You could also consider fund-raising yourself (if you have a just cause!), talking to local companies/Rotary/school/church organizations that you might have links with. Can you sublet your flat/bike/computer?

● Visa requirements

For most developing world countries, a tourist visa will suffice, however, an elective is often longer than a tourist visa and if anyone on the border finds out you are going to a hospital, they may well think you either need a work or a study visa. Explaining what an elective is can be difficult to a non-medic in a different language. It is therefore vital that you get the appropriate visa well in advance. Also consider that your passport should be valid for at least six months after your dates of travel.

PEARL OF WISDOM

Scan your passport, visa, occupational health documents and email them to yourself before leaving. Then, when your bags get nicked, you can always print off ID if there is an internet café.

● Your health, occupational health and immunizations

While one of the aims of your elective is to see conditions that are unusual back home, you should try not to catch them! Hence making sure you are up to date on your vaccines and having any additional ones is an early priority. It can take three months of repeated doses of some to build immunity, so don't leave this until the week before. You also need to consider appropriate antimalarials and, if you are working in an area of high HIV prevalence, **post-exposure prophylaxis** (normally available on deposit from your occupational health department) as well. Chemoprophylaxis currently comprises 4 weeks of Zidovudine and Lamivudine and for high risk cases or where drug resistance is suspected, a protease inhibitor (e.g. Nelfinavir or Indinavir).

⚡ HAZARD

If at all possible, try to get a summary sheet of your vaccines/medication on hospital-headed note paper in case of any problems. Impregnated nets are the best way of preventing being bitten and getting malaria. Don't swim in lakes as schistosomiasis (and hippos or crocodiles) are possibilities.

CLINICAL CONSIDERATIONS

Immunizations you might need

Visit www.fco.gov.uk for up-to-date recommendations:

    polio
    tetanus/diphtheria
    hepatitis A
    hepatitis B
    typhoid
    BCG
    rabies
    meningitis A and C
    Japanese encephalitis
    yellow fever

and consider:

    malaria prophylaxis (incl. Deet/net)
    HIV post-exposure pack

● Taking equipment/supplies

You may be asked to bring things with you. If this is a small amount, then you may be able to arrange it locally (though be very careful of taking any pharmaceuticals out with you). Always carry a letter from your hospital in your destinations language stating what they have asked for if you are taking anything yourself. Consider raising the money and using an organization such as Durbin (www.durbin.co.uk) to handle the logistics.

L) LEARNING POINTS

Packing

For you:

- books: (Oxford Handbooks, BNF, language/ guidebooks, light reading and diary)
- appropriate clothes (warm at night, cool during day, waterproofs and some smart wear. Do you need a white coat?)
- camera, torch, skipping rope, lock (and chain to attach bag to bus roof), first aid kit, sewing kit, MP3 player
- Do you need gloves etc (especially if you are latex allergic)
- Leave behind your valuables, and jewellery

For your destination:

- current newspapers/magazines if expats there. Little treats from home
- slightly out of date BNFs/textbooks for their library

● Indemnity

Most UK medical defence organizations (e.g. Medical Protection Society and the Medical Defence Union) will provide cover for students working in developing or resource-poor countries at no cost. It is well worth asking for them to provide a letter confirming this to save any problems when you arrive at your destination. (Note: This is not the case if you are doing an elective in the US, Canada or Israel.)

● Two other things to think about

1. **Environmental impact of travel** – In today's world, it is vital to consider the impact we have when travelling. Can you get to your destination without flying? If not, can you optimize everything else in your life? Consider carbon-offsetting (www.co2.org).
2. **Companies that organize your elective** – Organizing people's electives is now big business. The 'Package' elective can be bought off the shelf with very little thinking. The fact that you're reading this means that such an elective is probably not for you – and quite right too...the more you put in to doing the groundwork yourself, the more you will get out! Good on you!

● When you get back

Write about it and tell others – that way future students can gain the benefits from your discoveries and experience.

Making a career of it

Have you enjoyed your elective? Do you think this is something you want to continue to do? Once qualified, consider doing some courses and possibly the Diploma in Hygiene and Tropical Medicine or Diploma in the Medical Care of Catastrophes. Get clear in your mind why you are doing it and what you want to achieve. This can range from being the sole doctor in a remote village, to influencing public health on a global scale with the World Health Organization. In a lifetime, the two are by no means mutually exclusive. Spend an evening going through the World Health Organization's very comprehensive website to get a taste of such a career.

Summary

Your elective is a fantastic opportunity to experience healthcare in a different environment and, more importantly, get involved and hopefully contribute to a different culture. It needs extensive planning, though, to get the maximum out of it. Think about both the positive and negative impacts of your presence as you plan. For many people, their elective subsequently alters the rest of their careers.

FURTHER READING

Downloadable packs:

Preparing for your medical elective: Christian Medical Fellowship, HealthServe 5th Edition www.healthserve. org/files/medical_elective_fifth_edition.pdf

The Elective Pack from the International Health and Medical Education Centre, UCL www.ihmec.ucl.ac.uk/ ssc/electivepack.pdf

Book of hospitals and elective details:

Wilson M. *The Medic's Guide to Work and Electives around the World*. Arnold, London, 2009. ISBN 978-0-340-81051-4 www.medicstravel.org

Ethical issues:

Rethinking your elective Miranda and Finer, sBMJ Feb 2005; **13**: 45–48 http://student.bmj.com/issues/05/02/life/74.php

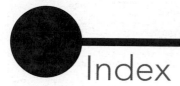

Index